Handbook of Ecotoxicology

Handbook of Ecotoxicology

Edited by **Giselle Tang**

FOSTER
ACADEMICS

New Jersey

Published by Foster Academics,
61 Van Reypen Street,
Jersey City, NJ 07306, USA
www.fosteracademics.com

Handbook of Ecotoxicology
Edited by Giselle Tang

© 2015 Foster Academics

International Standard Book Number: 978-1-63242-204-0 (Hardback)

Contents

Preface

Every book is a source of knowledge and this one is no exception. The idea that led to the conceptualization of this book was the fact that the world is advancing rapidly; which makes it crucial to document the progress in every field. I am aware that a lot of data is already available, yet, there is a lot more to learn. Hence, I accepted the responsibility of editing this book and contributing my knowledge to the community.

This book is completely based on ecotoxicology. It discusses the prospective aspects in this field. It discusses the genotoxicity of heavy metals in plants, chromatographic methodologies for the estimation of mycotoxin and effects of xenobiotics on benthic assemblages in different habitats. Laboratory findings of genotoxins on small mammals and bioindicators of soil quality and assessment of pesticides used in chemical seed treatments have also been described. There is also a comprehensive overview on European regulation REACH in marine ecotoxicology, X-ray spectroscopic screening for trace metal in invertebrates and alternative animal model for toxicity determination. This book is a well-organized and valuable collection of latest information on Ecotoxicology.

While editing this book, I had multiple visions for it. Then I finally narrowed down to make every chapter a sole standing text explaining a particular topic, so that they can be used independently. However, the umbrella subject sinews them into a common theme. This makes the book a unique platform of knowledge.

I would like to give the major credit of this book to the experts from every corner of the world, who took the time to share their expertise with us. Also, I owe the completion of this book to the never-ending support of my family, who supported me throughout the project.

Editor

Soil Ecotoxicology

Elke Jurandy Bran Nogueira Cardoso and Paulo Roger Lopes Alves
Universidade de São Paulo - Escola Superior de Agricultura "Luiz de Queiroz"
Brazil

1. Introduction

Expanding human activities have generated a mounting stream of waste, which is sometimes released into ecosystems at concentrations considered toxic for living organisms. As a result, populations of wild plants and animals are frequently exposed to toxic risks derived from the industrial wastes, pesticides, heavy metals, and other compounds that are released into the environment on a daily basis (Kappeler, 1979). These pollutants typically end up in soils, where potential toxic compounds come into direct contact with clays and organic material, which have a high capacity for binding to chemical compounds and substances (Bollag et al., 1992). Many organisms that live in soils, including beneficial soil fauna, are thus routinely exposed to high levels of pollution.

In these terrestrial ecosystems invertebrates and microorganisms drive a diverse array of biological and biochemical processes and play important roles in the carbon, nitrogen, phosphorus, and sulfur cycles by breaking down organic matter. Their transformation (mainly the mineralization) of organic material is broadly important for ecosystems and specifically important for agriculture, since the cycling of chemical elements provides much of plant's nutritional needs. Anthropogenic impacts, like the use of agricultural pesticides, can contaminate soils and thereby lead to an ecological imbalance in the soil community that may subsequently compromise the sustainability of the system (Cortet et al., 1999).

The study of the toxic effects that chemical substances have on living organisms, especially in the populations and communities of particular ecosystems, is the aim of the multidisciplinary field of ecotoxicology—a science that incorporates elements of ecology, toxicology, and chemistry, and explores the links between them (Römbke & Moltmann, 1996). Ecotoxicological tests aim to retrace the routes that pollutants take through the environment and to understand their interactions with it (Holloway et al., 1997).

In countries around the world, various such tests on soil organisms have been carried out for at least three decades (Spahr, 1981), in many cases using standardized soils and organisms in a laboratory setting (Organization of Economic Cooperation and Development [OECD], 1984a). Most ecotoxicological studies of soils are based on invertebrates and focus on worms, collembolans, or enchytraeids as bioindicators. The use of these groups has become standard because they are widely distributed, play important ecological roles, live in permanent contact with soils, reproduce quickly, and are easily maintained in laboratories (Edwards, 1989; Edwards et al., 1995; Römbke et al., 1996). The resulting body of research has succeeded in documenting a variety of negative effects that pesticides have on arthropods, microarthropods, and oligochaetes (Cortet et al., 2002; Jänsch et al., 2005b; Moser & Obrycki, 2009), as well as on soil microorganisms (Zhang et al., 2010).

2. The development of soil ecotoxicology

The growth of the human population, allied with technological advances and increasing consumption worldwide, have had adverse effects on the environment. The most worrisome repercussions are those that interfere with natural processes, and these are becoming more common. The impacts of human activities have mounted steadily since the industrial revolution in the eighteenth century, and by the twentieth century some irreversible and uncontrollable consequences for global environmental change and their destabilizing impacts on ecosystems had become apparent (Twardowska, 2004). Environmental disturbances are now capable of threatening the global environment, as shown by climatic changes and atmospheric pollution (Ramanathan et al., 2001), the qualitative and quantitative degradation of water and soil resources, and the severe impoverishment of biodiversity worldwide.

Given these developments, there is a mounting awareness that the very survival of humanity is dependent on current and future influences on environmental sustainability. Likewise, there is growing interest in understanding how the environment responds to sustained anthropogenic pressures, where man-made and natural pollutants end up in ecosystems, and what impacts they have there. Scientifically rigorous answers to these questions are urgently needed to develop the tools necessary to preserve a viable environment in the context of a growing human population (Twardowska, 2004).

The term "ecotoxicology" was coined in 1969 by R. Truhaut, who defined it as the scientific discipline that describes the toxic effects of various chemical agents on living organisms, and especially on populations and communities in ecosystems (Truhaut, 1977). Ecotoxicology is thus a blend of two different kinds of research: research on the natural environment (ecology), and research on the interactions of toxic chemical substances with individual living organisms (toxicology). Its links to chemistry, pharmacology, and epidemiology make it a truly multidisciplinary science that aims at understanding the origins and endpoints of chemical products in the environment (Connell et al., 1999). Present-day ecotoxicology encompasses a variety of scientific principles and methods capable of identifying and assessing the effects of substances released into the environment by mankind (Markert et al., 2003). It has evolved into a predictive science that aims to forecast the effects of potentially toxic agents on natural ecosystems and non-target organisms (Hoffman et al., 2003).

Ecotoxicology's obvious importance in environmental safety at both regional and global scales spurred the creation of a large number of organizations dedicated to environmental safety around the world. These include the International Academy of Environmental Safety (IAES) created in 1971, the International Society of Ecotoxicology and Environmental Safety (SECO-TOX) in 1972 and, in North America, the Society of Environmental Toxicology and Chemistry (SETAC) in 1979. In turn, the creation of these organizations called attention to the serious vacuum of useful scientific tools to guide decision-making regarding how to effectively regulate the release of pollutants into ecosystems (Twardowska, 2004).

In its early years, ecotoxicology developed more quickly for aquatic ecosystems than for terrestrial ecosystems. Water quality criteria were first defined by the United States

Environmental Protection Agency (EPA), which proposed benchmarks for analyzing leading pollutants and water quality attributes with the goal of broadening the use of hydrologic resources (for consumption, bathing, fishing, agriculture, and industrial uses) (Vighi et al., 2006). The European Inland Fisheries Advisory Commission (EIFAC), however, proposed that water quality criteria should focus on preventing impacts on any portion of the life cycle of fishes, preventing leaks from contaminated waterbodies, and, in addition, preventing the bioaccumulation of dangerous substances at levels dangerous to fish (Alabaster & Lloyd, 1978). As ecotoxicology matured for aquatic environments, the rise of internationally standardized methods and bioassays with invertebrates, fish, and algae generated a large database of toxicity for aquatic organisms long before such information existed for soil organisms (Van Straalen, 2002a).

In terrestrial ecosystems, despite a widespread recognition that soil invertebrates were functionally essential and useful as bioindicators of ecological disturbance (Schüürmann & Markert, 1997), until 1995 only two internationally accepted ecotoxicological methods were developed for soil organisms: a test using worms in artificial soils (OECD, 1984a) and an assessment method using plants (OECD, 1984b). Since then a broad assortment of new methods have appeared and the soil ecotoxicology database has grown impressively (Gomez-Eyles et al., 2009; Løkke & Van Gestel, 1998). Even so, the number of standardized tests available for the soil component of terrestrial systems is still lower than that available for aquatic systems.

Terrestrial ecotoxicology has been defined as the subfield of ecotoxicology which uses tests to study, evaluate and quantify the effects of toxic substances on the diversity and function in soil-based plants and animals (Garcia, 2004). Apart from measuring the relevant parameters and meeting environmental requirements, an effective toxicity test should be quick, simple, and replicable. A standard test should reveal a toxic response given variation in environmental conditions such as pH, solubility, exposure time, antagonism, and synergy. In this way, ecotoxicity tests can be classified in terms of exposure time (acute or chronic), observed effect (mortality, reduced growth, or compromised reproduction) or effective response (lethal or sublethal) (Kapanen & Itavaara, 2001).

The first stages of ecotoxicity analyses are carried out in the laboratory, where varying concentrations of the chemical products under study are added to an artificial substrate (International Organization for Standardization [ISO], 1999a, 1999b) or to natural soil (ISO, 2003), and acute toxicity, chronic toxicity, and behavioral effects are measured using soil quality bioindicators (Jänsch et al., 2005a).

Many bioassay methods have been developed to test acute toxicity (mortality) of chemical compounds, including local application, force-feeding, and immersion (Kula & Larink, 1997). However, standard international methods (OECD, 1984a; ISO, 1993, 1999a, 2004) are more broadly accepted. Most such tests are carried out using standard indicator organisms, but some authors have extrapolated and adapted the methods for other bioindicators (Förster et al., 2006; Jänsch et al., 2005b). While short-term tests of acute toxicity are useful for identifying highly toxic chemical compounds, they cannot determine whether organisms are more sensitive to those compounds during particular stages of their life cycles (Rida & Bouché, 1997). By contrast, medium-term tests of chronic toxicity measure the sublethal effects of harmful compounds on reproduction and growth, caused by biochemical and physiological disturbances (Hoffman et al., 2003). Standard tests of this kind have been established for some of the most commonly used non-target invertebrates in soil ecotoxicology, including collembola (ISO, 1999a), enchytraeids (ISO, 2004), and worms (OECD, 2004; ISO, 1998).

Since the duration of tests and the labor they require determine the costs of ecological risk assessments, it is sometimes preferable to obtain faster results using higher thresholds of sensitivity (ISO, 2008). For this reason avoidance tests, which provide a preliminary evaluation of contaminated soils in a short time, have increased in popularity (Natal-da-Luz et al., 2008) compared to toxicity tests. These tests are also ecologically relevant due to the high sensitivity thresholds, especially in assessments of remediated soils (Shugart, 2009), and are commonly used as a first triage tool to assess the habitation function of soils (Hund-Rinke et al., 2003), as they often provide results that other toxicity tests do not (Yearcley et al., 1996). Carrying out these tests in addition to acute and chronic toxicity tests can provide more detailed information on pollutants' impacts on organisms (Heupel, 2002), since changes in animal behavior can help quantify the effects of stress on individuals and populations (Markert et al., 2003).

The results of acute toxicity tests are expressed in values of LC_{50}, LC_x (lethal concentration), while those of chronic toxicity and avoidance tests are expressed in EC_{50}, EC_x (effective concentration), which indicates the concentration at which half of the study organisms die (LC_{50}) or the concentration at which a specific change in normal life parameters or behavior occurs (EC_{50}).

Ecotoxicological laboratory tests are a fundamental first tool for evaluating the ecological risks posed by polluted areas and remain commonly used (Bartlett et al., 2010; Correia & Moreira, 2010). However, exposure under laboratory conditions typically represents a worst-case scenario under which the effects on the organism are more severe than those observed in field conditions. This reflects the fact that the soil ecosystem is an extremely complex network of physical, chemical, and biological interactions, while laboratory tests are carried out in optimal conditions for growth and reproduction and thus ignore several variables that may play an important role in interactions between organisms and their environment. As this makes it difficult to extrapolate results from laboratory tests to field conditions (Van Gestel & Van Straalen, 1994), assessments of ecological risk should always seek to reproduce conditions in the field as closely as possible.

The first stages of ecotoxicological tests focus on individual species of the most important functional groups in the soil ecosystem (invertebrates and plants) (Garcia, 2004). The next stage aims to examine effects at the community level, using experiments in microcosms and mesocosms that incorporate multiple species and can provide more concrete results (Alonso et al., 2009). Microcosm tests (Figure 1) are generally carried out in the laboratory, where a few species of animals and/or plants are placed in natural soil. Mesocosm tests are large, multispecies systems that offer a high degree of environmental realism, since they are often carried out outdoors under natural light and rainfall conditions (Isomaa & Lilius, 1995). In a mesocosm test it is possible to study effects not only on individual species, but also at the population and community levels within an ecosystem (Crossland, 1994). These tests can identify cases in which impacts on a single species, whether a microorganism or a soil invertebrate, affect not just that species but the rest of the biota as well, potentially compromising entire ecosystems (Landis & Yu, 2004).

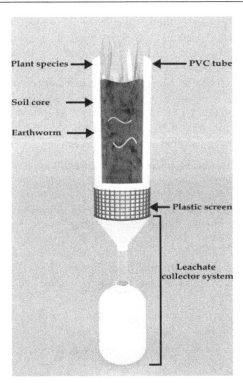

Fig. 1. Terrestrial Model Ecosystem (TME) used in the microcosms tests. On right side we represent the components of the TME, and on the left side, the ecological components. Adopted from Santos et al. (2011) (Virtual representation: Spisla, L. F.).

One drawback of the mesocosm model is the more challenging interpretation of results; in more complex systems it is harder to establish cause and effect between pollutant levels and degrees of community change, since many components of the system are dynamic and interdependent (Clements & Kiffney, 1994). Mesocosms assessments are also expensive and typically have few replicates, making them unviable for routine ecotoxicological triage (Crossland, 1994).

A third stage in environmental risk evaluations, considered the final step of this kind of analysis, involves measuring impacts in the field, under totally natural ecosystem and climate conditions. In this case, the observed responses reflect the effects of pollutants on soils with greater precision. Such tests may include analyses of bioaccumulation in animal tissues (Hoffman et al., 2003); the use of traps (pitfalls) (Querner & Bruckner, 2010) or soil samples (TSBF and Berlese funnels) to quantify the diversity and abundance of macro-, meso-, and microfaunal species (Anderson & Ingram, 1993; Araújo et al., 2010); litter bags (Förster et al., 2006) and bait-lamina tests (André et al., 2009) to measure the decomposition of organic material, in addition, direct (microbial biomass) and indirect (respirometry and enzyme tests) microbiological analyses may be used (Kapanen & Itävaara, 2001). Armed with this broad array of research tools for studying field conditions, it is possible to describe contaminated areas more precisely and to make more informed decisions, whether in the remediation or the prevention of environmental impacts.

In addition to the tests applied in the various stages of ecological risk assessments, new techniques and perspectives continue to enrich terrestrial ecotoxicology. One example are the genotoxicity tests with specific microorganisms, used to assess the impacts of waste products (Brown et al, 1991; Donelly et al, 1991). Other studies have documented important adaptive responses (genetics) following the exposure of living organisms to chemical products (European Centre for the Ecotoxicology & Toxicology of Chemicals [ECETOC], 2001; Lovett, 2000; Nota et al., 2010; Snape et al., 2004). This new subfield offers one more tool (molecular biology) for improving our understanding of environmental responses to toxic pollutants (Bradley & Theodorakis, 2002).

As noted previously, ecotoxicological tests are typically classified by their duration, the number of species involved (Landis & Yu 2004; Römbke et al., 1996), and further, subdivided along a gradient ranging from basic laboratory tests to complex field experiments (Figure 2). But while more complex tests offer more reliable information in ecotoxicological risk assessments, they have been used sparingly due to their complexity, cost, and long duration (Römbke & Notenboom, 2002). In general, terrestrial ecotoxicology has evolved towards ever more precise quantitative or qualitative assessments of the effects of pollutants in soils, as called for by numerous regulatory agencies worldwide as part of their efforts to determine acceptable concentrations of pollutants in soils, to limit their exposure, and to protect the terrestrial biota (Shugart, 2009).

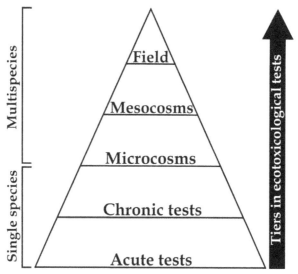

Fig. 2. Sequence of tiers used in Environmental Risk Assessment (ERA). From basic tests (acute) to most complex systems (field) of evaluation in soil ecotoxicology. According to the increases of tiers levels there is an increase of the bioassays complexicity and costs. Adapted from Landis & Yu (2004).

3. Bioindicators of soil quality

The term "soil health" has been defined by Pankhurst et al. (1997) as "the continued capacity of soil to function as a vital living system, within ecosystem and land-use boundaries, to sustain biological productivity, promote the quality of air and water environments, and maintain plant, animal, and human health". However, quantifying soil health with tools that track measurable properties of the system remains a steep challenge.

When measuring the health of a person or animal, one typically relies on parameters that describe the function of various organs, tissues, body fluids, physical structures (bones), and other components of the subject's body. In the same way, the living soil ecosystem is also composed of physical structures, chemical solutions, and biological communities in constant interactions that maintain vitality. Soils are a heterogeneous mix of biotic and abiotic components inhabited by a very complex community of organisms. The basic functions of the system depend on its structural and functional integrity, and this functionality is directly impacted by disturbances, needing some parameters for a better analysis (Edwards, 2004).

One appropriate way to quantify soil health is by measuring the parameters that make it a living system. Most attention in this regard has focused on indicators of the chemical and physical properties of the edaphic system, since biological properties are typically considered more difficult to predict or even measure. While a vast array of such indicators of soil quality or vitality have been proposed to date, it has become increasingly clear that biological indicators are needed to describe these dynamic systems (Blair et al., 1996). Biological processes may be more sensitive to soil changes than are indicators based on physical and chemical properties, which suggests that biological indicators could potentially offer early warnings of risks to ecosystems (Pankhurst et al., 1997).

Among the various definitions of the term "bioindication"(Heink & Kowarik, 2010), one that is widely accepted in terrestrial ecotoxicology describes it as a scientific analysis of field-collected ecological data with the aim of characterizing the environmental quality of a given area or region (Van Straalen, 1998). The same author emphasizes that bioindicator organisms should be directly or indirectly associated with the particular factor or suite of factors that they are intended to monitor. The utility of such biological indicators, also known as bioindicators or biomarkers, is that they describe the responses of living organisms exposed to or harmed by pollutants and thus provide information that can help prevent future damage to ecosystems (Hoffman et al., 2003). Biological indicators may thus be thought of as a barometer; just as barometers measure air pressure, the soil biota reflect the health of soils by revealing the cause of a particular effect or condition of the ecosystem (Van Straalen, 1998).

More than four centuries ago, long before the agricultural revolution, Vincenzo Tanara observed that soils are fertile when "birds such as ravens are attracted to a recently plowed field and scratch at the earth to eat the small invertebrates exposed by plowing". Much later, in the nineteenth century, Darwin argued that worms play an important role by building chambers in the soil profile and producing humus—which suggested that animals contributed directly to soil function (Paoletti et al., 1991). Since then, several studies have documented the importance of the soil biota for soil quality and vitality (Lavelle, 1996; Lavelle et al., 2006), and its potential for reflecting anthropogenic disturbances (Cortet et al., 1999; Paoletti et al., 1991; Van Straalen, 1998). By this measure, the first studies of bioindicators date to the beginning of the twentieth century. It is only more recently, amid mounting concern about the management and conservation of natural resources, that they have come to be regarded as important for assessing degraded environments (Paoletti et al., 1991).

In order to be considered promising biological indicators, organisms should occur in a variety of ecosystems, so that between-ecosystem comparisons are possible; should also be in contact with various stress factors, and thus interact with physical, chemical, and biological processes in soils; and should have direct functions and ecological importance in the edaphic system. Finally, a biological indicator should be easy and inexpensive to measure in order to facilitate sampling and experimentation, and be sensitive to a range of different management impacts, but not so sensitive that it vanishes altogether (Edwards et al., 1995; Stenberg, 1999).

Nowadays, bioindicators can be useful if a certain impact factor is not easily measurable. For example, in agricultural ecosystems the effects of pesticides such as the synthetic pyrethroid deltamethrin are easily observed in the epigeal invertebrate fauna, but the chemical determination of the residue is more difficult (Everts et al., 1989; Krogh, 1994). As toxicity tests are developed to help prevent immediate impacts of pollutants released into the environment, biomonitoring methods assess impacts over longer periods and track changing conditions in addition to the stressors or pollutants already present in the environment (Office of Environmental Health Hazard Assessment [OEHHA], 2008).

Invertebrate species that have shown potential as soil quality indicators include beetles (Kromp, 1999), ants (Lobry de Bruyn, 1999), spiders (Marc et al., 1999), mites (Koehler, 1999), collembolans (Cortet et al., 1999), enchytraeids (Didden & Römbke, 2001), nematodes (Yeates & Bongers, 1999), and worms (Blair et al., 1996; Paoletti et al., 1991; Paoletti, 1999). These invertebrates are used as inexpensive bioindicators, due to their ease of monitoring and the lack of restrictions on their use (Pankhurst et al., 1997). However, soil microorganisms can also offer valuable insights that can help interpret effects attributed to disturbance in terrestrial ecosystems (Bossio et al., 2005; Kapanen & Itävaara, 2001; Staley et al., 2010).

In an ideal world, all chemical products would be tested on every animal species before being released into the environment. As this is an unobtainable goal, representative species are used as triage tools in order to identify substances that are especially toxic. For soils, worms (*Eisenia* sp.), enchytraeids (*Enchytraeus* sp. and *Cognettia* sp.) and collembolans (*Folsomia sp.*) are the most widely used groups (Figure 3), due to their easy maintenance in laboratories and their relatively short generation times (Achazi et al., 1997; Fountain & Hopkin, 2005; Ronday & Houx, 1996).

There is a growing consensus among soil ecologists and farmers that worms may be one of the best indicators of soil quality (Doube & Schmidt, 1997). They are relatively easy to sample and identify, present in a broad variety of soils, regions, and climates, and indisputably important to food webs. Worms are important indicators of both soil quality and vitality, given that worm communities and their behavior are strongly affected by many leading agricultural practices such as crop plantation and rotation, fertilization, and the application of pesticides (Edwards, 2004).

Another important but less studied group in the subclass Oligochaeta are enchytraeids (Bardgett, 2005). While enchytraeids account for a small fraction of living biomass in soils, they are extremely important for nutrient cycling, feeding on fungal mycelium, rotting organic material, and associated microorganisms (Brussaard et al., 1990; Didden, 1993). They are considered "Key-species" for bioindication (Didden & Römbke, 2001; Römbke & Moser,

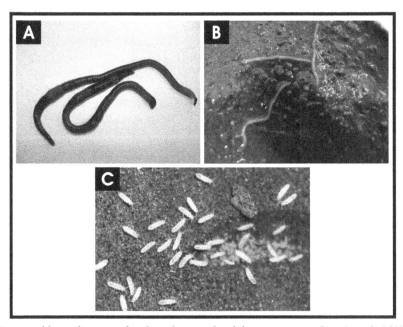

Fig. 3. Principal bioindicators of soil quality used in laboratory tests: *Eisenia andrei* (A); *Enchytraeus* sp. (B); *Folsomia candida* (C). (Photo: Ribeiro, C. M. & Santos, C. A.).

2002), especially in acidic soils (Didden, 1993), where they can replace worms as the functionally dominant soil fauna and where their abundance makes them good indicators under restricted conditions (Cole et al. 2002; Didden, 1993). Even so, while enchytraeids sometimes play an irreplaceable role in decomposition, they are less appropriate indicators than worms in more conventional soil conditions (Pankhurst et al., 1997).

The order Collembola is one of the most diverse and abundant groups of terrestrial arthropods on Earth, where they occur across all biomes (Coleman et al., 2004; Resh & Cardé, 2003;). A single square meter of dirt in temperate forest may contain more than 100,000 individuals (Anderson, 1978). While the direct effects of collembolans on ecosystem processes (like energy flows) may appear small due to their modest contribution to soil biomass and respiration (Coleman et al., 2004; Jänsch et al., 2005a), these organisms exercise significant influence on microbial ecology and soil fertility, since by feeding on dead organic matter and soil microorganisms they regulate decomposition and nutrient cycling processes (Culik & Zeppelini, 2003). The responses of these organisms to chemical products in the laboratory can thus be used to assess stress and inform legislative action concerning the ecological risks of certain substances (Van Straalen, 2002b).

Based on these foundations, the use of biological indicators of soil health and the process of assessing soil impacts have made considerable advances in recent years, as a large number of tests have used these model invertebrates to examine pesticide substances in soils and assess the risks they pose to the environment (Didden & Römbke, 2001; Gomez-Eyles et al., 2009; San Miguel et al., 2008).

4. Pesticides in soils

The term "pesticides" encompasses all active ingredients (a.i.) produced to control agricultural pests, independent of composition, formulation, and concentration. While the term is typically associated with substances that are used to control or kill pests (e.g., insecticides, fungicides, herbicides), it also applies to chemical compounds that alter pest behavior or physiology (e.g., insect repellents and growth regulators) (World Health Organization [WHO], 2010).

Synthetic insecticides and fungicides were developed after the Second World War and their application to crops spread quickly. Because insecticides were initially inexpensive and effective, farmers became dependent on the new tools, which soon replaced other chemical, cultural, and biological methods of pest control. The use of insecticides and fungicides in agriculture grew massively in the 1950s and 1960s and has continued to grow since; applying pesticides remains the leading method of pest and pathogen control today (Gulan & Cranston, 1994; Plimmer et al., 2003). Indeed, some studies on the benefits of pesticides have warned of the harm that could be caused by banning them, due to fears of a drop in agricultural productivity caused by pests (Delaplane, 2000; Walters, 2009).

Synthetic insecticides can be classified according to the presence or absence of carbon atoms, in its main molecule, as inorganic inseticides (e.g. boric acid) (Habes et al., 2006) and organo-synthetic insecticides. However, the organo-synthetic insecticides are considered the most important class of insecticides. They include the organochlorines, organophosphates, and carbamates, as well as a number of other classes like pyrethroids and neonicotinoids (Munkvold et al., 2006; Paulsrud et al., 2001). The first classes of fungicides included benzimidazoles, carboximides, morpholines, amino-pyrimidines, and organophosphorus compounds. In the 1970s there emerged a second generation of synthetic fungicides that included dicarboximides, phenylimides, triazoles, and fosetyl-aluminum. More recently developed fungicides include anilinopyrimidines, phenylpyrrole, and strobilurins, which show broad-spectrum action on the most common classes of pathogenic fungi (Plimmer et al., 2003).

In recent years the use of pesticides has increased in agriculture. Whether as a gas, a liquid, a powder, or in granulated form, these products remain commonly used to prevent or control pest outbreaks. One way in which pesticides are used to prevent pest outbreaks is by treating seeds with insecticides and fungicides. All commercially available corn and sorghum seeds are treated with fungicides, and some are also treated with insecticides (Lipps et al., 1988; Munkvold et al., 2006; Paulsrud et al., 2001). The practice is highly effective, offering significant reductions in pest damage (Giesler & Ziems, 2008; Lenz et al., 2008; Vernon et al., 2009). Treating seeds with insecticides has also become more common worldwide; in fact, a large proportion of the global increase in insecticides use is due to their increasing use on seeds (Hicks, 2000).

While the use of pesticides in agriculture provides benefits, it also has negative impacts, as evidenced by the increasing amounts of these chemical substances required year after year. It is well known that when pollutants come into contact with ecosystems they cause repercussions that can be traced from the molecular level up through tissues, organs, individuals, populations, and even entire communities (Schüürmann & Markert, 1997). Examples of the damage caused by pesticide wastes released into the environment include accidental poisoning of children and animals, intoxication of the people applying them, trace amounts in foods, phytotoxicity in plants, as well as soil, water, and air pollution (Dhingra, 1985; Paulsrud et al., 2001; Van Straalen, 2002b).

We have already discussed how the quality of terrestrial environments is compromised when non-target soil organisms are negatively impacted. Disturbances caused by pesticides in soils lead to qualitative and quantitative changes in the functioning of soils (Cortet et al., 1999), via two pathways. The first is via the direct contact of organisms with the substance, as is the case with pollinators, parasitoids, and beneficial predators, among others. The second way that organisms are negatively impacted is via the residues of these substances left on plants and elsewhere in the environment, which can harm the local fauna over longer time scales (Waxman, 1998).

Many insecticides kill target insects by acting on their nervous system. This specificity for the binding site of the substance also kills non-target organisms in the same way (Marrs & Ballantyne, 2004). Fungicides can harm non-pathogenic microorganisms (important in nutrient cycling) and antagonistic microorganisms (pathogen suppressors), thereby exercising a direct effect on disease control (Walters, 2009). In addition to insecticides and fungicides, herbicides are another class of pesticides with worrisome effects on the soil fauna. Developed to control weeds, they have shown harmful effects on macrofauna(Correia & Moreira, 2010), mesofauna (Heupel, 2002), and microorganisms (Widenfalk et al., 2008; Zhang et al., 2010).

Several studies to date have attempted to detect and assess the sublethal effects of pesticides on organisms exposed to contaminated soils. Bioassays have documented acute toxicity in the species *Eisenia fetida* exposed to fungicides in artificial soils (Anton et al., 1990), and under a variety of conditions (temperate and tropical climates). In tropical climates fungicides affect worms less severely than in temperate climates, perhaps due to the faster breakdown of pesticides in warm temperatures (Römbke et al., 2007). In addition to fungicides, studies have documented the impacts of insecticides (Gomez-Eyles et al., 2009) on the survival (Mostert et al., 2000), behavior (Capowiez & Berard, 2006) and even physiological processes (inhibition of cellulase activity) of worms in contact with contaminated soils (Luo et al., 1999). Severe population reductions of the collembolan *Folsomia candida* have also been documented in soils contaminated with insecticides (Cortet et al., 2002), but this effect is less apparent in field conditions, due to collembolans' propensity to avoid from contaminated areas. Collembola have also shown some degree of tolerance to some insecticides (San Miguel et al., 2008)

Herbicides used in agriculture also have impacts on worms (Heupel, 2002; Pereira et al., 2009). In tropical conditions, glyphosate and oxadiazon do not cause mortality in *E. fetida*. However, sublethal concentrations of these herbicides hamper the development of juvenile worms (Garcia et al., 2008). Other effects on worms in the presence of herbicides, such as population reductions and loss of body biomass, have also been documented (Stojanović et al., 2007).

In addition to the standard invertebrates typically used in terrestrial ecotoxicology tests, several other ecologically important organisms have been shown to suffer impacts from pesticides in soils (Kilpatrick et al., 2005). Examples include natural predators (Danfa et al., 2003; Moser & Obrycki, 2009) and invertebrate decomposers (Drobne et al., 2008;

Kreutzweiser et al., 2009; Niemeyer et al., 2006). There are also reports of significant reductions of microbial activity in soil (Malkomes, 1993), and it is known that bacteria numbers and fungal biomass are altered in pesticide-treated soils, perturbing decomposition processes and harming other organisms in the trophic chain (e.g., reducing the number of nematodes that feed on fungi) (Colinas et al., 1994; Ingham et al., 1991).

Thanks to the frequent use of these bioindicators in monitoring programs, it is now possible to determine which environmental changes occur when pesticides are exposed to terrestrial systems, with important implications for managing the early stages of pollution and for assessing the effectiveness of preventive or remedial measures taken to improve environmental quality (Van Straalen, 1998).

5. Case study: an ecotoxicological assessment of the pesticides used in chemical seed treatments

Treating seeds with chemicals is a common strategy for controlling pests and pathogens during the establishment of agricultural crops, since pesticides applied to the seed surface can repel and reduce the populations of insects and other organisms that attack seeds and seedlings (Baudet & Peske, 2006). In spite of these advantages, treating seeds with pesticides (e.g., fungicides, insecticides, and nematicides) can also have negative impacts, since it puts the a.i. of these substances in direct contact with soils, where soil organisms are exposed to them (Garcia, 2004).

Early studies of these xenobiotics' effects on soil organisms relied on standard tests with worms (*E. andrei*) and collembolans (*F. candida*), and demonstrated the potential of certain insecticides and fungicides for causing acute toxicity (OECD, 1984a; ISO, 1999a). In turn, the responses of these organisms in laboratory tests can be used to forecast, in a first tier, the environmental stresses that pesticides generate in the field (Van Straalen, 2002b).

Among the pesticides commonly used in chemical seed treatments, insecticides with the a.i. imidacloprid and fipronil have been studied via ecotoxicity tests on *F. candida* (San Miguel et al., 2008) and other collembolan species (Cortet & Poinsot-Balaguer, 2000; Heijbroek & Huijbregts, 1995; Peck, 2009). Reproductive impacts on the worm species *E. fetida* (Gomez-Eyles et al., 2009) and mortality on other oligochaete species (Mostert et al., 2002) have also been documented in the presence of these insecticides. Among the fungicides used to treat seeds, carboxin + thiram are known to have negative impacts on collembola (Larink & Sommer, 2002) and captan is known to affect worms (Anton et al., 1990).

The object of this study was to assess if pesticides (both fungicides and insecticides) used in chemical seed treatments affect the survival (acute toxicity) of *E. andrei* and *F. candida* in artificial soils.

5.1 Materials and methods

Methods for raising collembolans and worms were adapted from the ISO 11268-2 and ISO 11268-2 standards (ISO, 1998, 1999a). The organisms were raised and the bioassays carried out in a climate-controlled room where temperature measured 20 ± 2°C and illumination was set to a 12-hour cycle of light and darkness. The substrate typically used in terrestrial ecotoxicological tests is OECD artificial soil (OECD, 1984a); in this study we used a version of that substrate modified by Garcia (2004) and known as Tropical Artificial Soil (TAS), which includes powdered coconut fiber in its organic fraction.

We applied an aqueous solution containing the fungicides Captan® (captan - 480g of a.i. L^{-1}) and Vitavax® (38.7% carboxin + 37.5% thiram - 200g of a.i. L^{-1}), in addition to the insecticides Gaucho® (imidacloprid - 600g of a.i. L^{-1}) and Standak® (fipronil - 250g of a.i. L^{-1}), to the TAS immediately before starting the tests. Pesticide concentrations were established based on preliminary tests, and the control treatment was deionized water.

To assess mortality effects we carried out acute toxicity tests with E. andrei and F. candida (ISO, 1998, 1999a). For these tests, containers were filled with artificial soil treated (different volumes of soil for each organism) with the pesticide solution or with deionized water (control). At the start of the bioassay, 10 organisms (worms or collembolans) were added to each test container. Mortality was recorded by counting the number of adult organisms still alive after 14 days.

5.2 Results and discussion

Collembola (*F. candida*) suffered significantly higher mortality in TAS treated with the insecticides imidacloprid and fipronil compared to the control treatment (Figure 4). Mortality has previously been documented in this species following exposure to a low-concentration aqueous solution of fipronil for 96 hours (San Miguel et al., 2008). Likewise, imidacloprid, which is used in seed treatments, has been shown to reduce the abundance of the collembolan species *Onychiurus armatus* (Heijbroek & Huijbregts, 1995). It thus makes sense that soils where imidacloprid is present have reduced numbers of collembolans, possibly due to mortality (Peck, 2009).

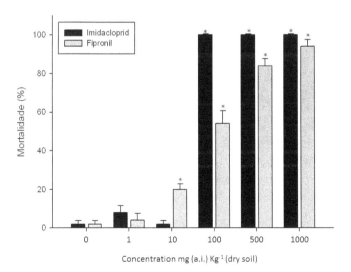

Fig. 4. Mortality (%) of *F. candida* in artificial soil treated with increasing concentrations of imidacloprid and fipronil (*P* < 0,05 on Dunnett´s test)

Fipronil acts on the insects' central nervous systems, where it inhibits a neurotransmitter responsible for regulating neuronal arousal. This neurotransmitter prevents the overstimulation of nerves, and its inhibition results in death. This mechanism of the insecticide's toxicity is mostly activated via ingestion, and is followed by spastic paralysis, death, and the elimination of sensitive insects (Coutinho et al., 2005). Since both the organisms and their food were in contact with contaminated soil in our study, it was very likely that the collembolans died due to inhibition of the neurotransmitter.

Imidacloprid also caused significant mortality in the worm species *E. andrei*, compared to the control treatment. Morphological alterations were also observed in these oligochaetes, which later died (Figure 5). Similar effects of mortality in *E. andrei/fetida* have been documented in studies of OECD artificial soil treated with imidacloprid (Buffin, 2003; Luo et al., 1999). While mortality of this worm species has been documented in polluted natural soils (Gomez-Eyles et al., 2009), effects in natural soils are typically weaker than those recorded in artificial soils, according to Kula and Larink (1997).

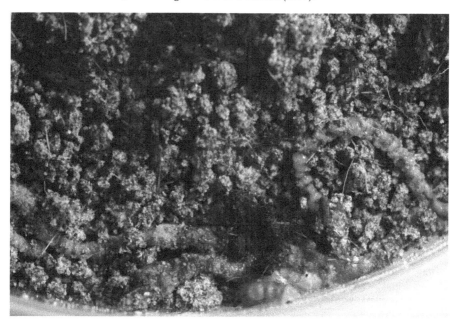

Fig. 5. Morphological alterations and mortality of worms (*E. andrei*) exposed to soils contaminated with the insecticide imidacloprid in an acute toxicity test. (Photo: Ribeiro, C. M.).

The lethal effect of imidacloprid on worms and collembolans may also be linked to blocked receptors in the nervous system. While insects are generally more susceptible to such blockage, which leads to the accumulation of acetylcholine (Buffin, 2003), this important neurotransmitter is present in many organisms and its blockage results in paralysis and sometimes death (Kidd & James, 1991). The worms that were in full contact with contaminated substrate for 14 days may have been affected in this way and subsequently died.

In addition to the insecticides, the fungicide captan also caused mortality in *F. candida*. In this case, however, the effect was only observed at high concentrations of the a.i. in the TAS. Mortality was not observed for worms exposed to captan, even at high concentrations. This result is corroborated by other studies that have shown that captan does not limit survival in these oligochaetes (Anton et al., 1990). Collembolan mortalities may be attributed to the compound tetrahydrophthalimide, a metabolite that is more common in captan (Reigart & Roberts, 1999) and which is responsible for the interaction of this fungicide, within cells, with the sulfhydryl, amino and hydroxyl groups of enzymes. These interactions are important because they may inhibit certain metabolic processes in the cells, leading to death (Waxman, 1998).

As in the test with the fungicide captan, we did not observe mortality of *E. andrei* exposed for 14 days to substrates treated with the pesticide carboxin + thiram. Worm mortality in the presence of fungicides has been previously reported in LUFA natural soil (ISO, 2003), in much lower doses than those in artificial soils (Röembke et al., 2007), which suggests that in our study the use of Artificial Tropical Soil may have partially buffered the negative effects of fungicides on worms.

In collembolans, significant mortality occurred in the presence of carboxin + thiram. In long-term studies, Frampton (2002) likewise documented declining collembolan abundance (and the total disappearance of some species) in agricultural soils treated with fungicides. This may be related to the mortality caused by the two fungicides examined in our study, and could furthermore indicate that collembolans are relatively sensitive to fungicides. There are few reports in the literature of the acute effects of carboxin + thiram on soil invertebrates. However, carboxin showed some impacts on and thiram was highly toxic to the aquatic organism *Daphnia magna* (EPA, 2004a, 2004b). It is possible that just one of the two substances in this product has negative impacts on collembolans. However, the concentration at which toxicity was observed was much higher than the calculated values for exposure to the fungicide in soils (data not shown). A similar conclusion was reached by Coja et al. (2006), who assessed the lethal effects of pesticides on *F. candida* and determined that the concentrations at which negative impacts were observed were higher than those found in soils, suggesting that they did not pose a threat in agricultural field conditions.

5.3 Conclusions

Artificial soils treated with the insecticides imidacloprid and fipronil, as well as the fungicides captan and carboxim + thiram, caused significant mortality in the collembola *Folsomia candida*. Only imidacloprid caused significant mortality in the worm *Eisenia andrei*.

6. References

Achazi, R. K., Chroszcz, G. & Mierke, W. (1997). Standardization of test methods with terrestrial invertebrates for assessing remediation procedures for contaminated soils. *Eco-Informa*, Vol. 12, (1997), pp. 284–89

Alabaster, J. S. & Lloyd, R. (1978). *Water Quality Criteria for Freshwater Fish*. Butterworths Scientific, ISBN 0408106735, London

Alonso, E., Nunez, M. G., Carbonell, G., Fernández, C. & Tarazona, J. V. (2009). Bioaccumulation assessment via an adapted multi-species soil system (MS.3) and its application using cadmium. *Ecotoxicological Environmental Safety*, Vol. 72, (May., 2009), pp. 1038–1044

Anderson, J. M. (1978). Inter and intrahabitat relationships between woodland cryptostigmata species diversity and diversity of soil and litter micro-habitats. *Oecologia*, Vol. 32, (1978), pp. 341–348

Anderson, J. M. & Ingram, J. S. I. (1993). *Tropical soil biology and fertility: A handbook of methods* (2nd ed.), Commonwealth Agricultural Bureaux (CAB) International, Wallingford.

André, A., Antunes, S. C., Gonçalves, F. & Pereira, R. (2009). Bait-lamina assay as a tool to assess the effects of metal contamination in the feeding activity of soil invertebrates within a uranium mine area. *Environmental pollution*, Vol. 157, No. 8-9, (Mar., 2009), pp. 2368-2377

Anton, F., Laborda, E. & Laborda, P. (1990). Acute toxicity of the fungicide captan to the earthworm *Eisenia fetida* (Savigny). *Bulletin Environmental of Contamination and Toxicology*, Vol. 45, (Jul., 1990), pp. 82-87, ISSN 0007-4861

Araújo, V. F. P., Bandeira, A. G. & Vasconcellos, A. (2010). Abundance and stratification of soil macroarthropods in a caatinga forest in northeast Brazil. *Brazilian journal of biology*, Vol. 70, No. 3, (Oct., 2010), pp. 737-46

Bardgett, R. (2005). *The Biology of Soil: A Community and Ecosystem Approach*. Oxford University Press, ISBN 0198525028, Oxford

Baudet, L. & Peske, S. T. (2006). A logística do tratamento de sementes, In: *Seed News* (Vol.10), Date of access 07/05/2011, Available from:
<http://www.seednews.inf.br/portugues/seed101/artigocapa101.shtml>

Bartlett, M. D., Briones, M. J. I., Neilson, R., Schmidt, O., Spurgeon, D. & Creamer, R. E. (2010). A critical review of current methods in earthworm ecology: From individuals to populations. *European Journal of Soil Biology*, Vol. 46, No. 2, (Dec., 2010), pp. 67-73, ISSN 1164-5563

Blair, J. M., Bohlen, P. J. & Freckman, D. W. (1996). Soil invertebrates as indicators of soil quality. In: *Methods for Assessing Soil Quality*, Doran, J. W. & Jones, A. J. pp. 273 – 291, Soil Science Society of America Special Publication, Vol. 49, Madison, WI.

Bollag, J. M, Myers, C. J. & Minard, R. D. (1992). Biological and chemical interactions of pesticides with soil organic-matter. *Science of the Total Environment*, Vol. 123, (Aug., 1992), pp. 205-217

Bossio, D. A., Girvan, M. S., Verchot, L., Bullimore, J., Borelli, T., Albrecht, A., Scow, K. M., Ball, A. S., Pretty, J. N. & Osborn A. M. (2005) Soil microbial community response to land use change in an agricultural landscape of western Kenya. *Microbial ecology*, Vol. 49, No.1, (Jan., 2005), pp. 50-62

Bradley, B. & Theodorakis, C. (2002). The post-genomic era and ecotoxicology. *Ecotoxicology*, Vol. 11, (Feb., 2002), pp. 7–9

Brown, K. W., Donelly, K. C. & Digiulio, D. G. (1991). Bacterial mutagenity of soil and water samples from Superfund site. *Nucl. Chem.*, Vol. 8, (1991), pp. 135-141

Brussaard, L., Bouwman, L. A., Geurs, M., Hassink, J. & Zwart, K. B. (1990). Biomass, composition and temporal dynamics of soil organisms of a silt loam soil under conventional and integrated management. *Netherlands Journal of Agricultural Science*, Vol. 38, (1990), pp. 283-302, ISSN 0028-2928

Buffin, D. (2003). Imidacloprid. *Pesticides News*, Vol. 62, (Dec., 2003), pp. 22-23

Capowiez, Y. & Berard, A. (2006). Assessment of the effects of Imidacloprid on the behavior of two earthworm species (*Aporrectodea nocturna and Allolobophora icterica*) using 2D terraria. *Ecotoxicology and Environmental Safety*, Vol. 64, (Jun., 2006), pp. 198–206

Clements, W. H. & Kiffney, P. M. Assessing contaminant effects at higher levels of biological organization. *Environmental Toxicology and Chemistry*, Vol. 13, (1994), pp. 357-359

Coja, T., Idinger, J. & Blumel, S. (2006). Effects of the benzoxazolinone BOA, selected degradation products and structure related pesticides on soil organisms. *Ecotoxicology*, Vol. 15, No.1, (Feb., 2006), pp.61-72

Cole, L., Bardgett, R. D., Ineson, P. & Adamson, J. (2002). Relationships between enchytraeid worms (Oligochaeta), temperature, and the release of dissolved organic carbon from blanket peat in northern England. *Soil Biology and Biochemistry*, Vol. 34, (Jan., 2002), pp. 599–607, ISSN 0038-0717

Coleman, D. C., Crossley, D. A. & Hendrix, P. F. (2004). *Fundamentals of Soil Ecology* (2nd ed.), Elsevier Inc., ISBN 0-12-179726-0, Athens, Georgia

Colinas, C., Ingham, E. & Molina, R. (1994). Population responses of target and nontarget forest soil organisms to selected biocides. *Soil Biology & Biochemistry*, Vol. 26, No.1, (Jan., 1994) pp. 41-47

Connell, D. W., Lam, P., Richardson, B. & Wu, R. (1999). *Introduction to Ecotoxicology: An introduction to electronic and ionic materials* (Vol. 4), Blackwell Publishing Ltd., ISBN 063203852-7,London, U.K.

Correia, F. V. & Moreira, J. C. (2010). Effects of glyphosate and 2,4-D on earthworms (Eisenia foetida) in laboratory tests. *Bulletin of environmental contamination and toxicology*, Vol. 85, No. 3, (Jul., 2010), pp. 264-268

Cortet, J., Gillon D., Joffre R., Ourcival J.-M. & Poinsot-Balaguer N. (2002). Effects of pesticides on organic matter recycling and microarthropods in a maize field: use and discussion of the litter-bag methodology. *European Journal of Soil Biology*, Vol. 38, (May., 2002), pp. 261-265

Cortet, J., Gomot-De Vauflery, A., Poinsot-Balaguer, N., Gomot, L., Texier, C. & Cluzeau, D. (1999). The use of invertebrate soil fauna in monitoring pollutant effects. *European Journal of Soil Biology*, Vol. 35, No. 3, (Jun., 1999), pp. 115-134

Cortet, J. & Poinsot-Balaguer, N. (2000). Impact of phytopharmaceutical products on soil microarthropods in an irrigated maize field: the use of the litter bag method. *Canadian Journal of Soil Science*, Vol. 80, No.2, (May., 2000), pp.237-249

Coutinho, C. F. B., Tanimoto, S. T., Galli, A., Garbellini, G. S., Takayama, M., Amaral, R. B., Mazo, L. H., Avaca, L. A. & Machado, S. A. S. (2005). Pesticides: Mode of Action, Degradation and Toxicity. Pesticides: *Ecotoxicol. and environment*, Vol. 15, (Dec.-Jan., 2005), pp. 65-72

Crossland, N. O. Extrapolation from mesocosms to the real world. (1994). *Toxicology and Ecotoxicology News*, Vol. 1, (1994), pp. 15-22

Culik, M. P. & Zeppelini, D. (2003). Diversity and distribution of Collembola (Arthropoda: Hexapoda) of Brazil. *Biodiversity and Conservation*, Vol. 12, (Jun., 1992), pp. 1119–1143, ISSN 0960-3115

Danfa, A., Amadou, B., Van Der Valk, H., Rouland, C., Mullié, W., Sarr, M. & Everts, J. (2003). Effects of chlorpyrifos and fipronil on soil macrofauna in a Sahelian savanna ecosystem. *Pesticides in non-target agricultural environments, environmental and economic implications - Joint European Southern African International Conference*, Cape Town, South Africa, Jan., 2003

Delaplane, K. S. (2000). *Pesticide Usage in the United States: History, Benefits, Risks, and Trends* (Bulletin 1121), Cooperative Extension Service of the University of Georgia College of Agricultural and Environmental Sciences, Georgia, U.S.A.

Dhingra, O. D. Importance and perspectives of seed treatment in Brazil. (1985). *Revista Brasileira de Sementes*, Vol. 7, No. 1, (1985), pp.133-138

Didden, W. & Römbke, J. (2001). Enchytraeids as Indicator Organisms for Chemical Stress in Terrestrial Ecosystems. *Ecotoxicology and Environmental Safety*, Vol. 50, (2001), pp. 25-43

Didden, W. A. M. (1993). Ecology of terrestrial Enchytraeidae. *Pedobiologia*, Vol. 37, (1993), pp. 2–29

Donelly, K. C., Brown, K. W., Andersson, C. S., Thomas, J. C. & Scott, B. R. (1991). Bacterial mutagenity and acute toxicity of solvent and aqueous extracts of soil samples from a chemical manufacturing site. *Environ. Toxicol. Chem.*, Vol. 10, (1991), pp. 1123-1131

Doube, B. M. & Schmidt, O. (1997). Can the abundance or activity of soil macrofauna be used to indicate the biological health of soils. In: *Biological Indicators of Soil Health*, Pankhurst, Doube, C. E. & Gupta, B. M., pp. 265-296, USSR, CAB International

Drobne, D., Blazic, M., Van Gestel, C. A. M., Leser, VOL., Zidar, P., Jemec, A. & Trebse, P. (2008). Toxicity of imidacloprid to the terrestrial isopod *Porcellio scaber* (Isopoda, Crustacea). *Chemosphere*, Vol. 71, No.7, (Apr., 2008), pp. 1326-1334

ECETOC - European Centre for the Ecotoxicology & Toxicology of Chemicals. (2001). *Document No. 42*, Brussels, Belgium

Edwards, C. A. (1989). Impact of herbicides of soil ecosystems. Plant Science, Vol. 8, (1989), p. 221-257

Edwards, C. A. (2004). *Earthworm Ecology* (Vol. 3), CRC Press LLC., Boca Raton, Florida

Edwards, C. A., Subler, S., Chen, S. K. & Bogomolov, D. M. (1995). Essential criteria for selecting bioindicator species, processes, or systems to assess the environmental impact of chemicals on soil ecosystems. In: *Bioindicator systems for soil pollution*, Van Straalen, N. M., Krivolutsky, D. A., pp. 67-84, Dordrecht: Kluwer

EPA - United States Environmental Protection Agency. (2004a) *Registration Eligibility Decision for Carboxin* (list A case 0012), EPA 738-R-04-015, Washington

EPA - United States Environmental Protection Agency. (2004b) *Registration Eligibility Decision for Carboxin* (list A case 0122), EPA 738-R-04-012, Washington

Everts, J. W., Aukema, B., Hengeveld, R. & Koeman, J. H. (1989). Side-effects of pesticides on ground-dwelling predatory arthropods in arable ecosystems. *Environmental Pollution*, Vol. 59, No. 3, (1989), pp.203-225

Förster, B., Garcia, M., Francimari, O. & Römbke, J. (2006). Effects of carbendazim and lambda-cyhalothrinon soil invertebrates and leaf litter decomposition in semi-field and field tests under tropical conditions (Amazonia, Brazil). *European Journal of Soil Biology*, Vol. 42, (Jul., 2006), pp. 171–179

Fountain, M. T. & Hopkin, S. P. (2005). *Folsomia candida* (Collembola): A "Standard" Soil Arthropod. Annu. Rev. Entomol. Vol. 50, (2005), pp. 201–222

Frampton, G. K. (2002). Long-term impacts of an organophosphate-based regime of pesticides on field and field-edge Collembola communities. *Pest Management Science*, Vol.58, No. 10, (Oct., 2002), pp. 991-1001

Garcia, M. V. B., Römbke J., Brito, M. T. & Scheffczyk, A. (2008). Effects of three pesticides on the avoidance behavior of earthworms in laboratory tests performed under temperate and tropical conditions. *Environmental Pollution*, Vol. 153, No. 2, (May. 2008), pp. 450-456

Garcia, M. V. B., (2004). Effects of pesticides on soil fauna: development of ecotoxicological test methods for tropical regions. *Ecology and Development Series* (No. 19), Zentrum für Entwicklungsforschung, University of Bonn, Germany

Giesler, L. J. & Ziems, A. D. (2008). *Plant Diseases Field Crops: Seed treatment fungicides for soybeans*, University of Nebraska–Lincoln Extension, Institute of Agriculture and Natural Resources, Nebraska, Lincoln

Gomez-Eyles, J. L., Svendsen, C., Lister, L., Martin, H., Hodson, M. E. & Spurgeon, D. J. (2009). Measuring and modelling mixture toxicity of imidacloprid and thiacloprid on *Caenorhabditis elegans* and *Eisenia fetida. Ecotoxicology and Environmental Safety*, Vol. 72, (Jan., 2009), pp. 71–79

Gulan, P. J. & Cranston, P. S. (1994). *The Insects: An outline of entomology*. Chapman & Hall, London

Habes, D., Morakchi, S., Aribi, N., Farine, J., & Soltani, N. (2006). Boric acid toxicity to the German cockroach, *Blattella germanica*: Alterations in midgut structure, and acetylcholinesterase and glutathione S-transferase activity. *Pesticide Biochemistry and Physiology*, Vol. 84, No.1, pp. 17-24

Heijbroek, W. & Huijbregts, A. W. M. (1995). Fungicides and insecticides applied to pelleted sugar-beet seeds - III. Control of insects in soil. *Crop protection*, Vol. 14, No. 5, (Aug., 1995), pp. 367-373

Heink, U. & Kowarik, I. (2010). What are indicators ? On the definition of indicators in ecology and environmental planning. *Environmental Monitoring and Assessment*, Vol. 10, (2010), pp. 584-593

Heupel, K. (2002). Avoidance response of different collembolan species to Betanal. *European Journal of Soil Biology*, Vol. 38, (May., 2002), pp. 273–276

Hicks, B. Leading the way in seed treatments. *Pesticide Outlook*, Vol. 11, (Aug., 2000), pp. 132–133

Hoffman, D. J., Rattner, B. A., Burton, G.A. & Cairns J. (2003). *Handbook of Ecotoxicology* (Vol. 2), Blackwell Scientific Publications, London, UK

Holloway, G. J., Crocker, H. J. & Callaghan, A. (1997). The effects of novel and stressful environments on trait distribution. *Functional Ecology*, Vol. 11, No. 5, (Oct., 1997), pp. 579-584

Hund-Rinke, K., Achazi, R., Römbke, J. & Warnecke, D. (2003). Avoidance test with *Eisenia fetida* as indicator for the habitat function of soils: results of a laboratory comparison test. *Journal of Soils & Sediments*, Vol. 3, No. 1, (2003), pp. 7–12, ISSN 1439-0108

Ingham, E. R., Parmelee, R., Coleman, D. C. & Crossley, D. A. (1991). Reduction of microbial and faunal groups following application of Streptomycin and Captan in Georgia no-tillage agroecosystems. *Pedobiologia*, Vol. 35, No. 5, (1991) pp. 297-304

ISO - International Organization for Standardization. (1993). *ISO-11268-1: Soil quality - Effects of pollutants on earthworms (Eisenia fetida)* (Part 1: Determination of acute toxicity using artificial soil substrate), Genève, Switzerland

ISO - International Organization for Standardization. (1998). *ISO-11268-2: Soil quality - Effects of pollutants on earth-worms (Eisenia fetida)* (Part 2: Method for the determination of effects on reproduction), Genève, Switzerland

ISO - International Organization for Standardization. (1999a). *ISO-11267: Soil quality - Inhibition of reproduction of Collembola (Folsomia candida) by soil pollutants*, Genève, Switzerland

ISO - International Organization for Standardization. (1999b). *ISO-11268–3: Soil quality – effects of pollutants on earthworms* (Part 3: Guidance on the determination of effects in field situations) Genève, Switzerland

ISO - International Organization for Standardization. (2003). *ISO 15799:2003: Soil quality - Guidance on the ecotoxicological characterization of soils and soil materials,* Genève, Switzerland

ISO - International Organization for Standardization. (2004). *ISO-16387: Soil quality - Effects of pollutants on Enchytraeidae (Enchytraeus sp.) - Determination of effects on reproduction and survival,* Genève, Switzerland

ISO - International Organization for Standardization. (2008). *ISO 17512-1: Soil quality - Avoidance test for determining the quality of soils and effects of chemicals on behavior* (Part 1: Test with earthworms *Eisenia fetida* and *E. andrei*), Genève, Switzerland

Isomaa, B. & Lilius, H. (1995). The urgent need for in vitro tests in ecotoxicology. *Toxicology in vitro,* Vol. 9, No. 6, (Dec., 1995), pp. 821-825

Jänsch, S., Amorim, M. J. & Römbke, J. (2005a). Identification of the ecological requirements of important terrestrial ecotoxicological test species. *Environ. Rev.,* Vol. 13, (Jun., 2005), pp. 51–83

Jänsch, S., Garcia, M. & Römbke, J. (2005b). Acute and chronic isopod testing using tropical *Porcellionides pruinosus* and three model pesticides. *European Journal of Soil Biology,* Vol. 41, (Oct., 2005), pp. 143–152

Kapanen, A. & Itävaara, M. (2001). Ecotoxicity tests for compost applications. *Ecotoxicology and environmental safety,* Vol. 49, No. 1, (Mar., 2001), pp. 1-16

Kappeler, T. (1979). The world ecotoxicology watch. *Environmental Science & Technology,* Vol. 13, No. 4, (Apr., 1979), pp. 412-415

Kidd, H. & James, D. R. (1991). *The Agrochemicals Handbook* (Third Edition), Royal Society of Chemistry Information Services, Cambridge, UK

Kilpatrick, A. L., Hagerty, A. M., Turnipseed, S. G., Sullivan, M. J. & Bridges, W. C. (2005). Activity of selected neonicotinoids and dicrotophos on nontarget arthropods in cotton: Implications in insect management. *Journal of Economic Entomology,* Vol. 98, No. 3, (Jun., 2005), pp. 814-820

Koehler, H. H. (1999). Predatory mites (Gamasina, Mesostigmata). *Agriculture, Ecosystems and Environment,* Vol. 74, (Jun., 1999), pp. 395-410

Kreutzweiser, D. P., Thompson, D. G. & Scarr, T. A. (2009). Imidacloprid in leaves from systemically treated trees may inhibit litter breakdown by non-target invertebrates. *Ecotoxicology and Environmental Safety,* Vol. 72, (May., 2009), pp. 1053–1057

Krogh, P. H. (1994). *Microarthropods as bioindicators,* PhD thesis, University of Arhus, Arhus, Denmark

Kromp, B. (1999). Carabid beetles in sustainable agriculture: a review on pest control efficacy, cultivation impacts and enhancement. *Agriculture, Ecosystems and Environment,* Vol. 74, (1999), pp. 187-228, ISSN 0167-8809

Kula, H. & Larink, O. (1997). Development and standardization of test methods for the prediction of sublethal effects of chemicals on earthworms. *Soil Biol. Biochem.,* Vol. 29, No. 3/4, (Mar.-Apr., 1997), pp. 635-639

Landis, G. W. & Yu, M. H. (2004). *Introduction to Environmental Toxicology: Impacts of Chemicals Upon Ecological Systems,* (3rd ed.), CRC Press Lewis Publishers, Boca Raton, FL.

Larink, O. & Sommer, R. (2002). Influence of coated seeds on soil organisms tested with bait lamina. European Journal of Soil Biology, Vol. 38, (Jun.-Dec., 2002), pp. 287–290

Lavelle, P. (1996). Diversity of soil fauna and ecosystem function. *Biol. Intern.,* Vol. 33, (Jul., 1996), pp. 3-16

Lavelle, P., Decaens, T., Aubert, M., Barot, S., Blouin, M., Bureau, F., Margerie, P., Mora, P. & Rossi J. P. (2006). Soil invertebrates and ecosystem services. *European Journal of Soil Biology*, Vol. 42, (Nov., 2006), pp. 3-15

Lenz, G., Costa, I. D., Zemolin, C. R., Karkow, D., Melo, A. A. & Silva, T. B. Phytotoxicity of fungicides applied on rice seeds (*Oryza sativa*). Revista da FZVA, Vol. 15, No.2, (2008), pp. 53-60

Lipps, P. E., Dorrance, A. E., Rhodes, L. H. & Labarge, G. (1988). *Seed Treatment* (Bulletin 638), The Ohio State University, Ohio

Lohry de Bruyn, I. A. (1999). Ants as bioindicators of soil function in rural environments. *Agriculture, Ecosystems and Environment*, Vol. 74, (Jun., 1999), pp. 425-441

Løkke, H. & Van Gestel C. A. M. (1998). *Handbook of Soil Invertebrate Toxicity Tests*.: John Wiley and Sons Ltd, Chichester, UK.

Lovett, R. L. (2000). Toxicologists brace for genomics revolution. *Science*, Vol. 289, (Jul., 2000), pp.53–57

Luo, Y., Zang, Y., Zhong, Y. & Kong, Z. (1999). Toxicological study of two novel pesticides on earthworm *Eisenia fetida*. *Chemosphere*, Vol. 39, No. 13, (Dec., 1999), pp. 2347-2356

Malkomes, H. P. Effect of pesticides used for seed treatment of potatoes on microbial activities in soil. Zentralblatt Fur Mikrobiologie, Vol. 148, n.7, p. 497-504, 1993.

Marc, P., Canard, A. & Ysnel, F. (1999). Spiders (Araneae) useful for pest limitation and bioindication. Agriculture, Ecosystems and Environment, Vol. 74, (Jun., 1999), pp. 229-273

Markert, B. A., Breure, A. M. & Zechmeister, H. G. (2003). *Bioindicators & Biomonitors: Principles, Concepts and Applications. Trace Metals and other Contaminants in the Environment*, (Vol. 6), Elsevier Science Ltd, Ann Arbor, Michigan

Marrs, T. C. & Ballantyne, B. (2004). *Pesticide Toxicology and International Regulation*, John Wiley & Sons, Ltd., Bradford, UK.

Moser, S. E. & Obrycki, J. J. Non-target effects of neonicotinoid seed treatments; mortality of Coccinellidae larvae related to zoophytophagy. *Biological Control*, Vol. 51, (Sep., 2009), pp. 487–492

Mostert, M. A., Schoeman, A. T. S. & Van Der Merwe, M. (2000). The toxicity of five insecticides to earthworms of the *Pheretima* group, using an artificial soil test. *Pest Management Science*, Vol. 56, No. 12, (Dec., 2000), pp. 1093-1097

Mostert, M. A., Schoeman, A. S., Van Der Merwe, M. (2002). The relative toxicities of insecticides to earthworms of the Pheretima group (Oligochaeta). *Pest Management Science*, Vol. 58, No.5, (Jan., 2002), pp. 446–450

Munkvold, G. P., Sweets, L. & Wintersteen, W. (2006). *Iowa Commercial Pesticide Applicator Manual. Seed Treatment*, Iowa State University, Ames, Iowa

Natal-Da-Luz, T., Römbke, J. & Sousa, J. P. (2008). Avoidance tests in site-specific risk assessment — influence of soil properties on the avoidance response of collembola and earthworms. *Environmental Toxicology and Chemistry*, Vol. 27, No. 5, (May., 2008), pp. 1112–1117

Niemeyer, J. C., Vilaça, D. & Da-Silva, E. M. Effects on *Cubaris murina* (Brandt) (Crustacea: Isopoda) biomass exposed to Glyphosate in the soil laboratory. *J. Braz. Soc. Ecotoxicol.*, Vol. 1, No. 1, (2006), pp.17-20

Nota, B., Verweij, R. A, Molenaar, D., Ylstra, B., Van Straalen, N. M. & Roelofs, D. (2010). Gene expression analysis reveals a gene set discriminatory to different metals in soil. *Toxicological sciences*, Vol. 115, No. 1, (Jan., 2010), pp. 34-40

OECD - Organisation for Economic Co-operation and Development. (1984a). *OECD - Guideline for Testing of Chemicals No. 207. Earthworm Acute Toxicity Test,* Paris

OECD - Organisation for Economic Co-operation and Development. (1984b). *OECD - Guideline for Testing of Chemicals No. 208. Terrestrial Plants, Growth Test,* Paris

OECD - Organization of Economic Cooperation and Development. (2004). *OECD - Guideline for Testing of Chemicals No. 222. Earthworm Reproduction Test (Eisenia fetida / andrei),* Paris

OEHHA - Office of Environmental Health Hazard Assessment. (2008). *Soil Toxicity and Bioassessment Test Methods for Ecological Risk Assessment: Toxicity Test Methods for Soil Microorganisms, Terrestrial Plants, Terrestrial Invertebrates and Terrestrial Vertebrates,* California Environmental Protection Agency, California, USA.

Pankhurst, C., Doube, B. M. & Gupta, V. V. S. R. (1997). *Biological Indicators of Soil Health,* CAB International, Cambridge

Paoletti, M., Favretto, M., Stinner, B., Purrington, F. & Bater, J. (1991). Invertebrates as bioindicators of soil use. *Agriculture, Ecosystems & Environment,* Vol. 34, No.1/4, (Feb., 1991), pp. 341-362

Paoletti, M. G. (1999). The role of earthworms for assessment of sustainability and as bioindicators. *Agriculture, Ecosystems and Environment,* Vol. 74, (Jun., 1999), pp.137-155

Paulsrud, B. E., Martin, D., Babadoost, M., Malvick, D., Weinzierl, R., Lindholm, D. C., Steffey, K., Pederson, W., Reed, M. & Maynard, R. (2001). *Oregon Pesticide Applicator Training Manual. Seed Treatment.* University of Illinois Board of Trustees, Urbana, Illinois

Peck, D. C. (2009). Long-term effects of Imidacloprid on the abundance of surface- and soil-active nontarget fauna in turf. *Agricultural and Forest Entomology,* Vol. 11, (Nov., 2009), pp. 405–419, ISSN 1461-9563

Pereira, J. L., Antunes, S. C., Castro, B. B., Marques, C. R., Gonçales, A. M. M., Gonçales, F. & Pereira, R. (2009). Toxicity evaluation of three pesticides on non-target aquatic and soil organisms: commercial formulation versus active ingredient. *Ecotoxicology,* Vol.18, (May., 2009), pp. 455–463

Plimmer, J. R., Gammon,D. W. & Ragsdale, N. N. (2003). *Encyclopedia of Agrochemicals* (Vol. 1-3), John Wiley & Sons, Inc., Hoboken, New Jersey

Querner, P. & Bruckner, A. (2010). Combining pitfall traps and soil samples to collect Collembola for site scale biodiversity assessments. *Applied Soil Ecology,* Vol. 45, No. 3, (Jul., 2010), pp. 293-297, ISSN 0929-1393

Ramanathan, V., Crutzen, P. J., Kiehl, J. T. & Rosenfeld, D. (2001). Aerosols, climate, and the hydrological cycle. *Science,* Vol. 294, No. 5549, (Dec., 2001) pp. 2119-2124, ISSN 1095-9203

Resh, V. H. & Cardé, R. T. Encyclopedia of Insects. (2003). *Encyclopedia of Insects* (1st ed.), Academic Press, San Diego

Reigart, J. R. & Roberts, J. R. (1999). *Organophosphate Insecticide - EPA 735-R-98-003, U.S. Environmental Protection Agency, Office of Prevention, Pesticides, and Toxic Substances: Recognition and Management of Pesticide Poisonings* (5th ed.), U.S. Government Printing Office, Washington, DC.

Rida, A. M. M. A. & Bouché, M. B. Earthworm toxicology: from acute to chronic tests. *Soil Biol. Biochem.,*Vol. 29, No. 3/4, (Set., 1997), pp. 699-703

Römbke, J., Bauer, C. & Marschner, A. (1996). Hazard Assessment of Chemicals in Soil. Proposed Ecotoxicological Test Strategy. *Environ. Sci. Pollut. Res.*, Vol. 3, (1996), pp. 78-82

Römbke, J., Garcia, M. VOL. B. & Scheffczyk, A. (2007). Effects of the fungicide benomyl on earthworms in laboratory tests under tropical and temperate conditions. *Archives of Environmental Contamination and Toxicology*, Vol. 53, (Nov., 2007), pp. 590-598, ISSN 0090-4341

Römbke, J. & Notenboom, J. (2002). Ecotoxicological approaches in the field. In: *Environmental Analycic of Contaminated Sitoo,* Sunahara, G. I., Renoux, A. Y., Thellen, C., Gaudet, C. L. & Pilon, A. John Wiley and Sons Ltd., Chichester, U.K.

Römbke, J. & Moltmann, J. F. (1996). *Applied Ecotoxicology.* CRC Lewis, Boca Raton, FL.

Römbke, J. & Moser, T. (2002). Validating the enchytraeid reproduction test: Organisation and results of an international ringtest. *Chemosphere*, Vol. 46, (Feb., 2002), pp. 1117-1140

Ronday, R. & Houx, N. W. H. (1996). Suitability of seven species of soil-inhabiting invertebrates for testing toxicity of pesticides in soil pore water. *Pedobiologia*, Vol. 40, (1996), pp. 106-12

San Miguel, A., Raveton, M., Lempérière G. & Ravanel, P. (2008). Phenylpyrazoles impact on *Folsomia candida* (Collembola). *Soil Biology & Biochemistry*, Vol. 40, (Sep., 2008), pp. 2351-2357

Santos, M. J. G., Ferreira, V., Soares, A. M. V. M. & Loureiro, S. (2011). Evaluation of the combined effects of dimethoate and spirodiclofen on plants and earthworms in a designed microcosm experiment. *Applied Soil Ecology*, Vol. 1528, (Apr., 2011), pp. 0-7, ISSN 0929-1393

Schüürmann, G. & Markert, B. (1997). *Ecotoxicology : ecological fundamentals, chemical exposure, and biological effects,* J. Wiley, New York

Shugart, L. R. (2009). *Emerging Topics in Ecotoxicology: Principles, Approaches and Perspectives,* Springer Science+Business Media, LLC., Oak Ridge, TN.

Snape, J. R., Maund, S. J., Pickford, D. B. & Hutchinson, T. H. (2004). Ecotoxicogenomics: the challenge of integrating genomics into aquatic and terrestrial ecotoxicology. *Aquatic toxicology*, Vol. 67, No. 2, (Apr., 2004), pp. 143-154

Spahr, H. J. The importance of collembola for soil biology and their suitability as test organisms for Ecotoxicology. (1981). *Anzeiger Fur Schadlingskunde Pflanzenschutz Umweltschutz*, Vol. 54, No. 2, (1981), pp. 27-29

Staley, Z. R., Rohr, J. R. & Harwood, V. J. (2010). The effect of agrochemicals on indicator bacteria densities in outdoor mesocosms. *Environmental microbiology*, Vol. 12, No. 12, (Dec., 2010), pp. 3150-3158

Stenberg, B. (1999). Monitoring soil quality of arable land: microbiological indicators. *Soil and Plant Science*, Vol. 49, (1999), pp. 1-24

Stojanović, M., Karaman S. & Milutinović, T. (2007). Herbicide and pesticide effects on the earthworm species *Eisenia fetida* (Savigny, 1826) (Oligochaeta, Lumbricidae). *Archives of Biological Sciences,* Vol. 59, No. 2, (2007), pp. 25-26, ISSN 0354-4664

Truhaut, R. (1977). Ecotoxicology: objectives, principles and perspectives. *Ecotoxicology and environmental safety*, Vol. 1, No. 2, (Sep., 1977), pp. 151-173

Twardowska, I. (2004). Ecotoxicology, environmental safety, and sustainable development--challenges of the third millennium. *Ecotoxicology and environmental safety*, Vol. 58, No. 1, (May., 2004), pp. 3-6

Van Gestel, C. A. M. & Van Straalen, N. M. (1994). Ecotoxicological test systems for terrestial invertebrates. In *Ecotoxicology of Soil Organisms,* Donker, M. H., Eijsackers, H. & Heimbach F., Lewis Publishers, Michigan, U.S.A.

Van Straalen, N. M. (1998). Evaluation of bioindicator systems derived from soil arthropod communities. *Applied Soil Ecology,* Vol. 9, (Sep., 1998), pp. 429-437

Van Straalen, N. M. (2002a). Assessment of soil contamination – a functional perspective. *Biodegradation,* Vol. 13, No. 1, (Jan., 2002), pp. 41–52, ISSN 0923-9820

Van Straalen, N. M. (2002b). Theory of ecological risk assessment based on species sensitivity distributions. In: *Species Sensitivity Distributions in Ecotoxicology,* Posthuma, L., Suter G. W. & Traas, T. P., Lewis Publishers, CRC Press

Van Straiten, N. M. & Van Gestel, C. A. M. (1993). Soil invertebrates and microorganisms. In: *Handbook of Ecotoxicology* (Vol. 1), Calow, P., Blackwell, Oxford, U.K.

Vernon, R. S., Van Herk, W. G., Clodius, M. & Harding, C. (2009). Wireworm management i: stand protection versus wireworm mortality with wheat seed treatments. *Journal of Economic Entomology,* Vol. 102, No. 6, (Dec., 2009), pp. 2126-2136

Vighi, M., Finizio, A. & Villa, S. (2006). The evolution of the environmental quality concept: from the U.S. EPA red book to the european water framework directive. *Environmental science and pollution research international,* Vol. 13, No.1, (Jan., 2006), pp. 9-14, ISSN 0944-1344

Walters, D. (2009). *Disease Control in Crops - Biological and Environmentally Friencly Approaches,* Blackwell Publishing Ltd., Edinburgh, U.K.

Waxman, M. F. (1998). *Agrochemical and Pesticides Safety Handbook.* Lewis Publishers, Boca Raton, FL.

WHO - World Health Organization. (2010). *The who recommended classification of pesticides by hazard and guidelines to classification,* Stuttgart, Germany

Widenfalk, A., Bertilsson, S., Sundh, I. & Goedkoop, W. (2008). Effects of pesticides on community composition and activity of sediment microbes e responses at various levels of microbial community organization. *Environmental Pollution,* Vol. 152, (Apr., 2008), pp.576-584

Yearcley, R. B., Lazorchak, J. M. & Gast, L. C. (1996). The potential of an earthworm avoidance test for evaluation of hazardous waste sites. *Environmental Toxicology and Chemistry,* Vol. 15, No. 9, (Feb., 1996), pp. 1532–1537, ISSN 0730-7268

Yeates, G. W. & Bongers, T. (1999). Nematode diversity in agroecosystems. *Agriculture, Ecosystems and Environment,* Vol. 74, (Jun., 1999), pp.113-135

Zhang, C., Liu, X., Dong, F., Xu, J., Zheng, Y. & Li, J. (2010). European Journal of Soil Biology Soil microbial communities response to herbicide 2,4-dichlorophenoxyacetic acid butyl ester. *European Journal of Soil Biology,* Vol. 46, No. 2, (Mar., 2010), pp. 175-180

2

Contribution of X-Ray Spectroscopy to Marine Ecotoxicology: Trace Metal Bioaccumulation and Detoxification in Marine Invertebrates

Sabria Barka

Research Unit of Marine and Environmental Toxicology, UR 09-03, University of Sfax,
Institut Supérieur de Biotechnologie de Monastir,
Tunisia

1. Introduction

Among contaminants involved in pollution, metals are peculiar as they are natural components of the geosphere. Volcanic eruptions, soil leaching, anthropogenic inputs, constitute different sources of metal introduction in the aquatic environments, the sea being the final receptacle for toxic compounds (Ramade, 1992). Moreover, they are the only environmental pollutants that are nor made nor degraded by Men but that are transported and transformed in various products that affect living organisms. Metals are present in the sea within its different compartments: water column, sediments and in marine biota, where they are accumulated from water or food. Some metals are so essential to living organisms that when their availability is limited, the process of life development may be negatively affected. In fact, beyond a given threshold, all metals, whether essential or not, may have toxicological and ecotoxicological effects. Toxic effects may impair numerous biological and physiological processes, leading to animal death and threatening of species conservation. The energy costs associated with excreting and/or detoxifying the ingested/assimilated metals may decrease growth and reproduction with negative consequence on population density and on ecological intra and inter-specific relations.

Aquatic organisms accumulate metals to concentrations several folds higher than those in the surrounding medium (Bryan, 1979; Rainbow et al., 1990). However, metal bioaccumulation per se is not necessarily an indication of adverse effects (Campbell & Tessier, 1996) and knowledge of the physiological processes of accumulation and detoxification is needed to understand the significance of accumulated trace metal concentrations in marine animals collected from contaminated areas, especially in the frame of biomonitoring programs (Rainbow, 1993; 1997). Metal bioaccumulation in organisms is a natural physiological process or a consequence of an accidental surcharge. In both cases, common cellular structures involved in metal sequestration are requested (Jeantet et al., 1997). Cells have various biological ligands, such as metalloproteins, to which metals can bind, on the one hand, and their organites (ie lysosomes, endoplasmic reticulum) are involved in metal sequestration (Ballan-Dufrançais, 1975; Brown, 1982; Mason & Jenkins, 1995; Nott & Nicolaidou, 1989a; Simkiss & Taylor, 1995; Raimundo et al., 2008; Simkiss & Masson, 1983). Total metal body burden may reflect the presence of inert particles mineralized (the so-called granules) within tissues and cells which are no longer involved in metabolism. Generally, metal bioaccumulation studies in marine invertebrates give quantitative data on the tissular partitioning of metals (organotropism) but few of them consider the physico-chemical form in which metals are present within tissues or cells. However, these informations would improve our knowledge on cellular mechanisms involved in metal sequestration, storage and excretion as those mechanisms neutralize the toxicity of metals and could then be considered as detoxification processes.

The presence of metals in granules has been evidenced in marine invertebrate cells by microanalytical techniques (Nott, 1991). These techniques have been currently used in the field of geology, mineralogy, petrology, paleontology, environmental atmospheric analysis, marine chemistry etc. Although their applications are increasing in material sciences, such as semiconductors, thin film, nanoparticles and surfaces (Van Cappellen, 2004), these techniques have been rarely used in the field of biological sciences even if it is currently used in medical science since 1995 and particularly in toxicology (George, 1993; Börjesson & Mattsson, 2004).

The aims of this chapter are to present the potential use of X-Ray spectroscopy as an analytical tool in biological systems and its possible applications (combined with ultrastructural studies) in the field of ecotoxicology, while highlighting its important contribution to understand how marine invertebrates cope with environmental metals.

2. Trace metal bioaccumulation in marine invertebrates

Metals are naturally present in seawater in very low concentrations (Bruland, 1983). Major metals (Sodium, Magnesium) are present in an order of mmol Kg^{-1}; minor metals (Lithium, Barium) in µmol to nmol Kg^{-1} and trace metals (Copper, Zinc, Mercury, Cadmium, Lead) in pmol Kg^{-1}. Metals are also present in sediments and in benthic biota (Bryan & Langston, 1992; Rainbow et al., 2011). Marine invertebrates are continuously exposed to variable concentrations of trace metals in seawater. There is a huge intra and inter-specific variability in metal accumulation among marine invertebrates. Metal accumulation occurs to different extent in individuals depending on the metal, its speciation, its bioavailability, and the considered species and biotic (body size, gender, molting, reproductive and developmental stage, and feeding habit…) and abiotic (temperature, salinity, pH…) factors (Marsden & Rainbow, 2004; Wang & Rainbow, 2008).

2.1 Background metal concentration

Metal concentrations in marine invertebrates collected from different natural areas show a considerable variation even in close phylogenetically related species (Table 1). As for essential metals, they are accumulated to fulfill metabolic requirement. Various proteins, enzymatic or not, require metals to be functional. The blood of marine invertebrates may contain respiratory pigments which bind to copper or iron. For example, annelids X-Ray microanalysis revealed the presence of Fe, Ca and small amounts of Zn. *Tubifex* hemoglobin also contained Cu and Pb (Rokosz & Vinogradov, 1982). The elemental mapping of several biological structures showed that different metals may also have a structural role as they can be constitutive of annelid jaws (Bryan & Gibbs, 1980; Gibbs & Bryan, 1980), crab cuticule (Schofield et al., 2009) or copepod exoskeleton (unpublished data). In fact, metals which are essential for metabolic requirement can be theoretically estimated (Depledge, 1989; Pequegnat et al., 1969; White & Rainbow, 1985) and is necessary to identify these components when interpreting total essential metal concentration in invertebrate tissues or bodies or to identify a metal deficiency (Rainbow, 1993).

However, non essential metals such as silver or cadmium were also found in molluscs and crustaceans collected in non-polluted areas (Ballan-Dufrançais et al., 1982; Bustamante, 1998; Martoja et al., 1985; & Pétri, 1993). Their presence in animals could not be explained.

This illustrates the concept of metal background concentration which is considered as the typical metal concentration found in invertebrates collected from a habitat remote from anthropogenic inputs of metals (Rainbow, 1993). Evaluating background concentrations is necessary when invertebrates, collected from metal polluted areas, are used as biomonitors to know if metal concentrations have risen over a baseline in order to make realistic interpretations of the metal content in animals

2.2 Metal accumulation patterns

Aquatic invertebrates are able to cope with the pollution pressure of their environment due to the existence of different adaptive strategies which have been reviewed, for instance, by Mason and Jenkins (1995):

- they are able to limit the entrance of the contaminant into their body;
- they are able to balance uptake by an increased excretion, the total concentration in the organisms remaining constant;
- they are able to detoxify and store the metals which have entered the organism.

From and ecotoxicological point of view, and considering the fate and transport of metals in the marine environment, understanding metal uptake and excretion in invertebrates is important as these organisms may be exposed to very high levels of metals.

Experimental metal exposure of marine invertebrates, particularly well studied crustaceans, showed that these animals have developed different pattern of metal accumulation which vary within and between invertebrates depending on the metal and the species (Rainbow, 1998, 2002, 2007).

The first pattern, currently described in palaemonid decapod crustaceans, consists of a balance of the rate of zinc excretion to that of zinc uptake resulting in a regulation of this metal as its body concentration is maintained relatively constant (Rainbow, 1993, 1997; White & Rainbow, 1984). In many decapod species of crustaceans, it has been well established that essential metal concentrations remain steady over a large range of metal concentrations in their medium. This pattern has been described in numerous crustacean species not only for Zn but also for Cu (Amiard et al., 1987; Maranhaño et al., 1999; Rainbow, 1993, 1998; Sandler, 1984). Some exceptions have been mentioned such as the absence of Cu regulation in the freshwater shrimp *Macrobrachium malcomsonii* (Vijayram & Geraldine, 1996) or of Zn regulation in crabs *Uca annulipes* and *U. triangulis* (Uma & Prabhakara, 1989). In other classes of crustaceans (amphipods, copepods...), Zn and Cu regulation processes are generally absent (Amiard et al., 1987; Barka et al., 2010; Chen & Liu, 1987; Clason et al., 2003; Rainbow, 1988; Rainbow & White, 1989; Zauke et al., 1996) even if the amphipods *Allorchestes compressa* and *Hyatella azteca* appear to be able to control their internal metal content (Ahsanullah & Williams, 1991; Borgmann et al., 1993).

Taxon	Class	Species (geographical zone)	Cu	Zn	Ni	Cd	Hg	Reference
Crustaceans	Copepod	*Tigriopus brevicornis* (North Atlantic coast)	9	66	9.3	0.17	0.34	(Barka *et al.*, 2010)
		Calanus hyperboreus (Greenland Sea)	4.7 5.6	80 104	11.4	4.0 0.75	0.31	Pohl (1992) Ritterhoff & Zauke (1997b)
		Euchaeta barbata (Greenland Sea)	4.5	225	3.9	0.16	0.27	Ritterhoff & Zauke (1997b)
		Acartia clausi (Méditerranean)	55	1270		0.6		Zarifopoulos & Grimaris (1977)
		Metridia longa (Greenland Sea)	7.5	351	19.7	0.71	0,68	Ritterhoff & Zauke (1997b)
	Isopod	*Ceratoserolis trilobitoides* (Gould Bay) (Elephant island)	38 46	40 40				De Nicola *et al.*, 1993
		Idotea baltica males (Bay of Naples, Italy)		292		0.68		
	Barnacle	*Capitulum mitella* (Cape d'Aguilar, Honk Kong)	29.2					Phillips & Rainbow, 1988
		Amphibalanus amphitrite Algeciras Bay (Spain)	94-225	852-4170	2.7-26			Morillo *et al.*, 2008
	Amphipod	*Platorchestia platensis* Hoi Ha Wan, Honk Kong Cape d'Aguilar, Honk Kong		199 193		fl		Rainbow *et al.*, 1989
		Orchestia gammarellus Whithorn, Scotland Girvan, Scotland	132 66					Rainbow *et al.*, 1989
	Branchiopod	*Daphnia magna* (Lab culture, from Huo Qi Ying Bridge, China)	230					Fan *et al.*, 2011
	Decapod	*Systellaspis debilis* (Deep Sea North East Altlantic)				12		Ridout *et al.*, 1989
Molluscs	Bivalve	*Mizuhopecten yessoensis* (Peter the Great Bay, Japan) Digestive gland Kidney				142 11.6		Lukyanova *et al.*, 1993
		Mizuhopecten magellanicus (US Atlantic coast) Digestive gland Kidney				94 62.6		Uthi & Chou, 1987

Table 1. Mean metal concentration in marine invertebrates collected from natural marine areas ($\mu g.g^{-1}$ dry weight of total body or organ when indicated).

Contribution of X-Ray Spectroscopy to Marine Ecotoxicology: Trace Metal Bioaccumulation and Detoxification
in Marine Invertebrates

29

In fact, metal accumulation can be modelled at a given exposure by a straight line, the slope of each line representing the accumulation rate (μg Metal g^{-1} d^{-1}) at that exposure. By plotting these rates against the exposure concentration, we can calculate the slope of this line which is the metal accumulation index (μg g^{-1} d^{-1} per μg L^{-1}, or L g^{-1} d^{-1}) (according to Rainbow & White, 1989). From this index, it is possible to calculate the expected accumulated concentration at any exposure concentration at any exposure time. Sometimes, in the case of the lack of significant change in animal body metal concentration over controls, the calculation of accumulation index helps to decide whether a true metal regulation is occurring or not (when the index is very low).

When metal exposure concentration is high, regulation breakdowns and the excretion rate fails to match the uptake rate, resulting in a net increase in body metal. Therefore, metals may remain in metabolically available form, without detoxification, thus exerting a toxic effect after metabolic requirement is fulfilled. Another possible route for metal is to remain in detoxified form such as mineralized granules. In both cases, metal excretion may occur in a different form, metabolically available and detoxified, depending on the considered component.

Amphipods have a low zinc uptake rate with no significant excretion, resulting in a weak accumulation of this metal (Rainbow & White, 1989). Conversely, barnacles (*Elminius modestus*) (Rainbow, 1987; Rainbow & White, 1989) strongly accumulate zinc, in detoxified granules, with no excretion. Net accumulation strategies were reported for crustaceans from polar regions with respect to Pb and Cu in Arctic zooplankton *Calanus hyperboreus*, *Calanus finmarchicus*, *Metridia longa*, *Themisto abyssorum* (Ritterhoff & Zauke, 1997a,d) and to Co, Cu, Ni, Pb, and Zn in the Antarctic copepods *Calanoides acutus* (Kahle & Zauke, 2002a) and *Metridia gerlachei* (Kahle & Zauke, 2002b).

3. Localization of metals in marine invertebrates

Invertebrates possess several mineral bioaccumulation structures in various organs. Bioaccumulation structures were first revealed empirically or with imperfect histochemical techniques (Ballan-Dufrançais, 2002). In 1815, Brugnatelli observed "shalky structures" in malpighian tubules (involved in mineral homeostasis) of silk worms using microchemical techniques. Ever since, literature reported the existence of metal-containing granules in invertebrates, whether these were exposed or not to trace metals. Numerous studies have shown that metal-containing granules occur in many different aquatic phyla (from protozoa to arthropoda) (Ballan-Dufrançais, 1975; Barka, 2007; Mason & Jenkins, 1995; Moore, 1979; Nassiri et al., 2000; Simkiss & Mason, 1983; Nott, 1991; Viarengo & Nott, 1993; Vogt & Quinitio, 1994).

3.1 Bioaccumulation structures in invertebrates: size, aspect, composition and role

Due to their chemical composition (Masala et al., 2002) and their different stages of development, metal granules are highly variable in form, composition, size, aspect and location (Brown, 1982; Mason & Jenkins, 1995; Roesijadi & Robinson, 1994). Sectioned granules show different types of internal structure. It may be homogeneous (Walker, 1977), diffuse (Mason et al., 1984), conglomerated (Isheii et al., 1986; Reid & Brand, 1989), crystalline (Masala et al., 2002) or arranged in concentric strata (Ballan-Dufrançais, 1975; Hopkin & Nott, 1979; Pigino et al., 2006). Their size is about less than a μm to several μm.

Depending on their elemental composition, cytochemical and chemical characteristics granules have been classified into three types (Brown, 1982 and references cited therein):

i. Fe-containing granules in which Fe may be present in ferritin (Brown, 1982; Hopkin, 1989; Viarengo & Nott, 1993). They are generally amorphous but crystalline structures have already been observed in copepods, , isopods, molluscs and amphipods (Barka, 2000; Jones et al., 1969; Quintana et al., 1987; Moore, 1979 respectively) (Fig. 1);

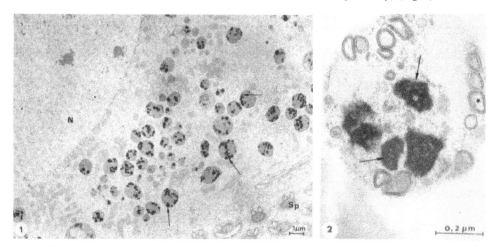

Fig. 1. (1) Ultrastructure of the ovotestis of *Planorbarius*, at the last stage of vitellogenesis.The platelets (P) of the oocyte contain electron-dense of ferritin (arrows), N, nucleus, Sp, cross section of the sperm tails. Unstained osmicated ultrathin sections. X 7800. (2) Detail of a snail platelet. Natural occurence of crytalline form of ferritin (arrows). Unstained non-osmicated section. X 50 000 (after Quintana et al., 1987).

ii. Cu-containing granules also contain S and small amounts of Ca, K, P, Cl and Fe. Cu-rich granules have been observed in the digestive tract of many crustaceans living in pristine areas (Al-Mohanna & Nott, 1987; Barka, 2007; Hopkin & Nott, 1979; Nassiri et al., 2000; Walker, 1977). Vogt and Quinitio (1994) found Cu-rich granules in hepatocytes of *Penaeus monodon*. Weeks (1992) and Nassiri et al. (2000) have also observed Cu-rich granules in the ventral caeca of the Amphipod *Orchestia gammarellus*. The same type of granule was found in the midgut of control and Cu-exposed marine isopods (Tupper et al., 2000) and in the digestive cells (sometimes in the apex) of copepods (Barka, 2007)(Fig.2a).

Ag was also found in Cu-S rich granules in control and Ag exposed crustaceans, (Barka 2007; Chou et al., 1998)(Fig.2b).. This may be explained by the fact that both metals, belonging to the group I.b of the transition elements, display many similar chemical properties as suggested by Hogstrand and Wood (1998) and Bury et al. (2003). Ag is probably naturally bioaccumulated which may indicate that these granules are not simply a sink for essential metals. Silver is often found in the aquatic environment in the 1-100 ng.l^{-1} range and known to avidly bind to inorganic and organic ligand (Kramer et al., 2002). It is interesting to notice that larger Cu-containing granules were found in animals inhabiting Cu-contaminated environments (Barka, 2007; Brown, 1982). There is a great variability in the morphology

Contribution of X-Ray Spectroscopy to Marine Ecotoxicology: Trace Metal Bioaccumulation and Detoxification in Marine Invertebrates

31

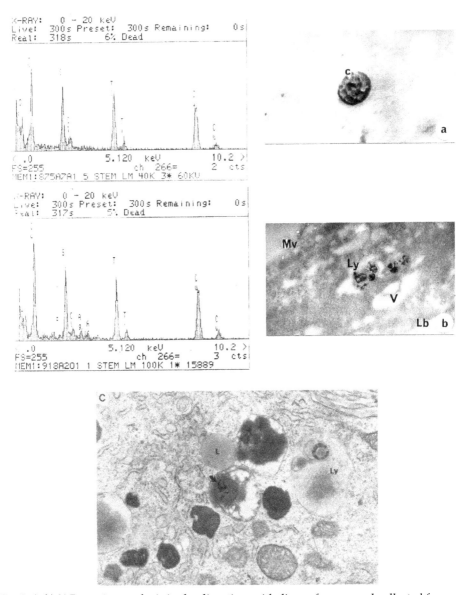

Fig. 2. (a,b) X-Ray microanalysis in the digestive epithelium of a copepod collected from an clean area. (a) Occurrence of Cu and S in a compact granule (c). x 29 000 (b) occurrence of Cu, P, S and Ag in the fine granular material of a lysosome (Ly), (Lb) basal lamina, (Mv) microvilli, (V) vacuole. x 19 000 (after Barka, 2007). (c) Bivalve (*Abra alba*) collected from Morlaix Bay, France. Ultrastructural aspect of a digestive cell, showing voluminous lysosomes (Ly) with vacuoles containing a flocculent material and electron dense particles (arrow). L, lipidic inclusion. Microanalysis revealed the presence of Si, Fe, Cu, P, Zn and S. X 26 000 (after Martoja et al, 1988).

of the different Cu-containing granules. However, they are all usually homogeneous, spherical structures with no concentric structuring;

iii. Ca-containing granules which may be of two types based on their composition:
   * Ca carbonates granules, of a high purity are found in arthropod and gastropod conjunctive tissues as they are involved in Ca storage. They play no role in heavy metal physiology - although Pb may substitute to Ca2+ (George, 1982). They are generally big (several μm) and have a typical aspect, with concentric strata. These particular structures, also called calcospherites or spherocrystals, have been found in the digestive cells of different terrestrial and aquatic arthropods (Ballan-Dufrançais, 2002; Barka, 2007; Corrêa et al., 2002; Defaye et al., 1985; Durfort, 1981) (Fig. 3);

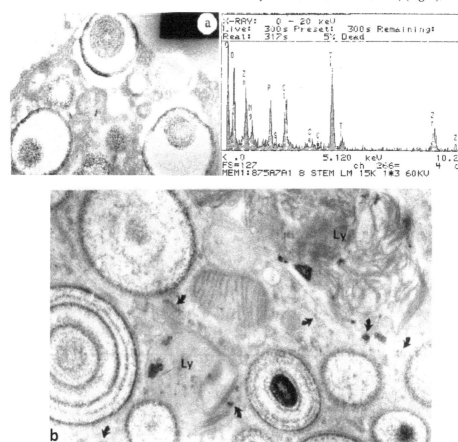

Fig. 3. (a) Occurrence of Zn, Mg, P, S and Ca in spherocristals (2–2.5 lm) in digestive epithelium of a benthic copepod collected from the North Atlantic french coast. Note the dark and light concentric strata. x ·14,000 (after Barka, 2007) (b) Coackroach (*Blatella*) exposed to CH₃HgCl through diet for 4 days. Ultrastructural aspect of ileum. Note the abundance of spherocristals. Microgranules of Hg, Zn and Cu (arrows) are present in lysosomes (Ly) and in the endoplasmic reticulum. x 40 000 (after Jeantet, 1981).

Contribution of X-Ray Spectroscopy to Marine Ecotoxicology: Trace Metal Bioaccumulation and Detoxification in Marine Invertebrates

33

- Ca phosphate granules in which Ca is present together with Mg, but also other metals such as Al, Ag, Ba, Co, Fe, Mn, Pb, Sn et Zn; and possibly Cu, Cd, Cr, Hg and Ni (Roesijadi & Robinson, 1994). They are intra and inter-specifically highly variable in aspect and composition which depend on environmental metal concentration (George, 1982; Sullivan et al., 1988) (Fig. 4). They are generally small (less than 1 μm) although huge ones (10-15 μm) have been found in marine bivalves (Marsh & Sass, 1985).

The precise role of these particular granules still remains unclear but the literature reported two major functions: regulation of storage and release of Ca^{2+} and detoxification (Corrêa et al., 2002; Simkiss & Wilbur, 1989; Simmons et al., 1996). These granules may act as a calcium reservoir serving as a source of calcium for metabolic needs, maintaining Ca homeostasis, exosqueleton replacement after moulting as suggested for crabs (Becker et al., 1974) or building material of skeletal tissue in molluscs (Jacob et al., 2011). However, several authors proposed a metal detoxification role for Ca granules (Mason & Simkiss, 1982; Simkiss, 1981). Furthermore, calcium granules, whose formation being controlled by factors associated with ion fluxes as evidenced by Masala et al. (2002), could act as a passive sink for toxic metals during calcium precipitation.

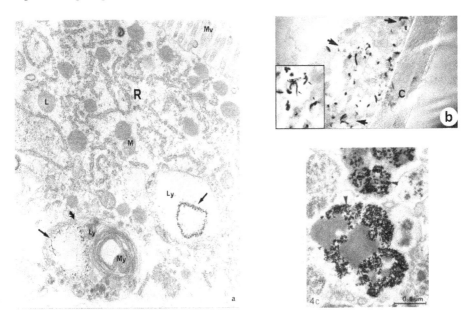

Fig. 4.(a) Ultrastructural aspect of a digestive epithelium cell of a benthic copepod exposed to Hg. Occurrence of dense granules (arrows) in lysosomes (Ly), L, lipids, Lu, lumen, M, mitochondria, Mv, microvilli, My, myelin. x 15 000. (b) Occurrence of Cu, S and Ag in needles (arrows) in lysosomes of the integument of Ag exposed copepods. x 19 000 and x 72 000 for detail (after Barka, 2007) (c) Scallop (*Pecten maximus*) collected from the Channel coast. The lysosomes of the digestive gland contain dense granules (arrows) in which numerous elements are detected (Cd, Ag, Mo, Br, Zn, Cu, Fe, Ca, S, Si, Al). x 48 600 (after Ballan-Dufrançais et al., 1985).

3.2 Localization of metals in tissues and cells

Depending on the species, metal granules have been observed in different tissues. In gastropod mollusks, granules have been found in different tissues such as the digestive gland (Mason & Nott, 1981), gills (Marigomez et al., 1990; Mason et al., 1984; Simkiss & Mason, 1983), gonads (Quintana et al., 1987) and conjunctive tissue (Bouquegneau & Martoja, 1982; Martoja et al., 1980; Martoja et al., , 1985;). In crustaceans, these structures have been found in the digestive tract (Bernard & Lane, 1961; Guary & Négrel, 1981; Hopkin & Nott, 1979, 1980; Vogt & Quinitio, 1994) and in the cuticular hypodermic parenchyme (Barka 2007; White, 1978 as cited in Mason & Jenkins, 1995). Actually, metal granules are present in almost every invertebrate tissues particularly in those involved in digestion and/or excretion (Mason & Jenkins, 1995).

At the cellular level, metal granules occur in the cytoplasm of cells and more specifically in the basal lamina, or cell apex and within specific organelles such as endoplasmic reticulum (ER) Golgi complex, Golgi vesicles and even in nucleus. Granules can also occur in the paracellular space or in the digestive lumen.

3.3 Origin and formation of metal mineralized structures

Metals entering cells may have different possible intracellular routes which have been summarized in Fig. 5.

X-Ray microanalysis associated with transmission electron microscopy showed that metal granules were found in vesicles originated from the lysosomal system. Granule elemental composition showed the presence of different minerals associated with C, S, O which have an organic origin. Cu-granules elemental composition showed the coexistence of Cu and S suggesting that sulphur may be the chelating agent. Heavy metals, especially class"b" metals, tend to form stable complexes with the sulphydryl residues of amino acids and polypeptides. Metallothionein, with its high cysteine content, and other metal-binding proteins, are sulphur donors to which Cu can bind. Degraded proteins are finally engulfed into lysosomes where they are digested. This pathway has been extensively described in the literature and explains the presence of metals in lysosomes (Mason & Jenkins, 1995; Viarengo & Nott, 1993). As some metals can induce metallothioneins, it is reasonable to think that the presence of Cu (associated with S), Hg or Cd in lysosomes results from the breakdown products of metal-thionein that might be turning over at high rates in metal exposed animal. However, Cu-granules may also be a consequence of respiratory pigment catabolism as suggested by Moore & Rainbow (1992) in amphipods although, Cu in lysosomal granules may have entered the organelle through an ATPase transport system localized on the lysosomal membrane as found in lobster hepatopancreatic cells (Chavez-Crooker et al., 2003).

In Ca phosphate granules, lipofuscin may be the organic matrix for metal incorporation within lysosomes as it has been shown for Cd and Zn which passively adsorb onto lipofuscin (George, 1983b). Over time, some lysosomes fit together and/or evolve into voluminous heterolysosomes in which cytoplasmic material is progressively mineralized. Heterolysosomes then get smaller, more condensed and filled with indigestible products and finally they mature into residual bodies (also called tertiary lysosomes) in which enzyme activities are exhausted. The great variability of granules may be due to these different development stages.

Contribution of X-Ray Spectroscopy to Marine Ecotoxicology: Trace Metal Bioaccumulation and Detoxification
in Marine Invertebrates

35

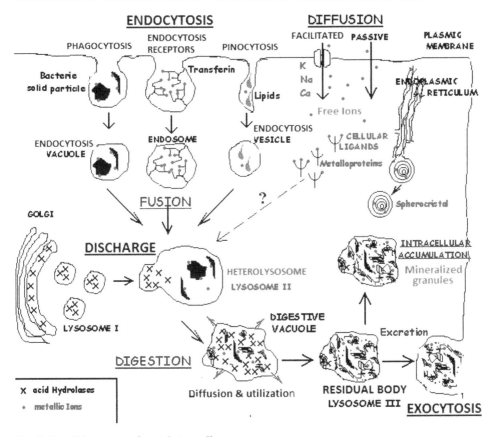

Fig. 5. Possible routes of metals in cells.

The structure of calcospherites granules is concentric and are thought to have a different origin. They may be derived from the endoplasmic reticulum (Ballan-Dufrançais, 2002; Cheung & Marshall, 1973; Corrêa et al., 2002). Studies based on cytochemical assays found a phosphatase activity associated to calcospherites, which strengthened the hypothesis that the reticulum is involved in the formation of these structures (Corrêa et al., 2002; Loret & Devos, 1995).

The mechanism of granule intra and extracellular growth was shown to be different from that leading to their initial formation. Metal accretion onto granules has been observed *in vivo* and *in vitro* (George, 1983a, b; Simkiss, 1981). Concentric strata have been interpreted as alternated period of accretion and resorption (Carmichael et al., 1979). In lysosomes, pH variations facilitate metal adsorption onto granule surfaces in sites where Ca dissociated during dissolution (Taylor et al., 1988) or following Mg^{2+} loss (Nott & Nicolaidou, 1989b).

Overall, the precise elemental composition of granules using microanalytical techniques would greatly improve our understanding of the origin and the formation process of metal granules and, indirectly, metal handling mechanisms in invertebrates.

3.4 Technical considerations: ultrastructure and microanalysis

3.4.1 Technique principle

Energy dispersive X-Ray Microanalysis in Transmission Electronic Microscopy (EDMA-TEM) consists of an analytical TEMs which is equipped with detectors for sample analysis. It works similarly to TEM: the sample is bombarded with an electron beam, emitting x-rays at wavelengths characteristic to the elements being analyzed. The elemental composition and abundance may be determined.

In the following section, technical considerations concerning Energy dispersive X-Ray Microanalysis connected with Transmission Electronic Microscopy are presented.

3.4.2 Sample preparation before analysis

The specimen-preparation technique influences the elemental data generated by granule microanalysis. Animal or tissue glutaraldehyde fixation was found to remove chemical elements such as Cd, as shown by the study of Nott and Langston (1989) who found Cd in granules in Cd-exposed molluscs when they used a cryo-preparation method instead of a chemical one. The original work of Vesk and Byrne (1999) on mussels, showed that chemical fixation and sectioning influenced elemental distribution and concentration of metals in granules. Furthermore, the conservation of tissues in a basic medium (sodium cacodylate) prior to dehydratation do not favour the preservation of cytoplasmic bioaccumulation structures (Ballan-Dufrançais, 1975).

Resin embedding composition must be known. In general, resins contain chloride and an important Cl peak appears among those of other elements in microanalysis spectra.

As for grids, on which embedded specimens are deposited, they should be made of a metal that is not suspected to be found in biological tissues. Titanium grids rather than copper or gold grids are preferable.

Sample section thickness must be chosen to fit the best resolution. TEM samples should be thin enough to be beam transparent and resolve morphological detail using the transmitted electron signal. X-Ray spatial resolution depends on thickness sections because the energy beam, commonly between 100kV - 400kV in the analytical TEM, should not be destructive to samples. However, X-Ray generation is low for thin samples as the ionization volume is small but when analyzing thicker samples, absorption corrections (material density and thickness) should be made to minimize electron scattering.

3.4.3 Advantages and inconvenient

X-ray microanalysis of thin specimens in the Transmission Electron Microscope (TEM) offers nano-scale information on the chemistry of materials. X-Ray microanalysis is a non destructive, sensitive, accurate and precise technique. It is qualitative and semi-quantitative. However, quantitative results can be obtained from the relative x-ray counts at the characteristic energy levels for the sample constituents. The spectra obtained are easy to interpret.

The inconvenient, besides the fact that the instrument is expensive and requires technical skills, is that X-ray signals (peaks) for some elements may interfere with those for non-

Contribution of X-Ray Spectroscopy to Marine Ecotoxicology: Trace Metal Bioaccumulation and Detoxification
in Marine Invertebrates

37

biological elements (grid, resin…), which make the interpretation difficult. The sensitivity threshold of the technique can also be considered as a limiting factor. When metal concentration is too low, it remains undetectable. Furthermore, the thickness of the non-osmicated specimen section does not allow a proper visualization of the elements located, in the tissue or cell. Generally, when TEM is used, even if metal granules are visualized at the ultrastructural level, these structures do not necessarily match microanalysis data. This is due to the fact that X-Ray microanalysis and TEM observation require different preparation for each specimen (non-osmicated/thin section versus osmicated/ultrathin section)

4. Ecotoxicological significance of metal bioaccumulation

Crustaceans exoskeleton, molluscs shell etc are likely to come into contact with the surrounding metals and to bind to them before these are absorbed. When ingested (via food or water), metals entering the gut or passing through permeable membranes (e.g. gills), are absorbed in soft tissues where they are stored or excreted. Metals accumulated in soft tissues are likely to be present in two phases: dissolved in the cytoplasm, mainly as complexes with metal-binding proteins, or incorporated in metal-rich granules (Mason & Jenkins, 1995). All metals have the potential to be deleterious to cellular mechanisms, even though some of them are essential to normal metabolic processes. The metal accumulation levels, and consequently the potential toxicity, cannot be predicted only on the basis of concentration in water or in tissues (Simon et al., 2011). It is the only bioavailable fraction that is potentially toxic and of ecotoxicological relevance (Rainbow 1998, 2002, 2006). Therefore, toxicity cannot be attributed to the global body/organ metal burden but depends on the physico-chemical form in which the metal is present in organisms. From an ecotoxicological perspective/point of view, partitioning of metals (soluble versus insoluble) is important as metals, within these two fractions, are involved in different metal handling mechanisms and may have different mobility from prey to predator species through trophic transfer.

4.1 Metal detoxification

Lysosomal systems are ubiquitous in all invertebrate cells, particularly well developed in digestive and excretory cells. Furthermore, the occurrence of increasing lysosomes in metal exposed animals, compared to controls, leads to think that these organelles are involved in metal cellular responses. Two major metal storage pathways have been reported in invertebrates, namely, cytosolic metalloproteins and/or the lysosomal system (Amiard et al., 2006; Marigomez et al., 2002; Mason & Jenkins, 1995; Rainbow, 2006; Viarengo & Nott, 1993). The complexation of metals by metallothioneins (MTs), non-enzymatic metalloproteins, is one mechanism used by the invertebrate cell to prevent the activation of toxic metals in the cytoplasm (Viarengo et al., 1987). Consequently, in addition to their role in homeostasis, MTs have often been considered as detoxification proteins, although this latter function is still open to debate (Cosson et al., 1991).

The great ability of invertebrates to accumulate metals in granules probably enables these animals to cope with the presence of (potentially dangerous levels of) metals in their surroundings and to be protected from their toxicity (Brown, 1982; Desouky, 2006; Masala et al., 2004; Mason & Jenkins, 1995; Mason & Nott, 1981; Simkiss & Mason, 1983; Stegeman et al., 1992). In some species, these concretions remain in the cell for a relatively long period of time before they are excreted (Fowler, 1987; Sullivan et al., 1988; Nott, 1991). Actually granules were found in the digestive lumen of the crab *Callinectes sapidus* (Becker et al., 1974; Guary & Negrel, 1981) and of the copepod *Tigriopus brevicornis* (Barka, 2007) suggesting that metal detoxification occurs (if the release of granules into the lumen is followed by an excretion in the gut)(Fig. 6). In fact, the dissolution of mineralized granules may occur along the digestive tract as showed in a terrestrial arthropod by Krueger et al. (1987). The decrease of the pH of lumen contents from distal to proximal regions of the digestive tract appears to be a major effector of granule dissolution. These authors also studied the effect of pH on the dissolution of isolated granules *in vitro*. They showed that the release of calcium, phosphorus, and magnesium from granules increased exponentially as the pH of the bathing medium was decreased. Loss of structural integrity of the granules accompanied mineral release and also increased as pH of the bathing medium was lowered *in vitro*. This study suggests that, during gut transit, metals can be released from granules for both prey and predators.

The significant increase in the number of granules upon exposure to metals and the fact that they are generally insoluble and associated with digestive or excretory tissues (i.e., digestive gland, hepatopancreas, kidney, among others) and, consequently, can be excreted, may give further evidence for their role in detoxification (Desouky, 2006; Marigomez et al., 2002; Pullen & Rainbow, 1991; Simkiss, 1976; Simkiss & Taylor, 1989).

4.2 Biomagnification and trophic transfer

Many authors have suggested that the subcellular distribution of metals is critical for metal assimilation in predators (Amiard-Triquet et al., 1993; Nott & Nicolaidou, 1990; Reinfelder & Fisher, 1994; Wang & Rainbow, 2000). If we consider invertebrates as prey species, it is important to know how metals are distributed in animals because physicochemical characteristics of these contaminants (in prey species) control their mobility and thus their transfer to the next trophic level. Furthermore, accumulated metal in prey that is trophically available to one predator is not necessarily equally trophically available to another predator feeding on the same prey, given the variability between invertebrate digestive systems (Rainbow & Smith, 2010). The literature provides evidence that the assimilation of trace elements in predators is governed by the cytoplasmic distribution in prey (Ni et al., 2000; Nott & Nicolaidou, 1993; Reinfelder & Fisher, 1991, 1994; Wallace & Lopez, 1996 , 1997; Wallace et al., 1998;).

Metals, mainly present in the fraction operationally described as the soluble fraction, are probably more able to be transferred along a food chain than those in insoluble fractions. Consequently, detoxification processes based on metallothioneins presumably would not protect the consumer since these proteins can be degraded, in predator gut, during digestion. Incorporation of metals into detoxified granules may lead to a "transfer of metal detoxification along marine food chains" since such inorganic compounds may not be assimilated during gut passage in the predators. The fact that metals can strongly bind to pre-existing granules, should guaranty a minimal remobilization. Consequently, metal incorporation, in detoxified form, within granules should reduce metal toxicity to the next trophic level although Khan et al., (2010) showed that cadmium bound to metal rich granules from an amphipod caused oxidative damage in the gut of its predator. These findings suggest that granules, largely considered as having limited bioavailability, may as also be toxic to some extent.

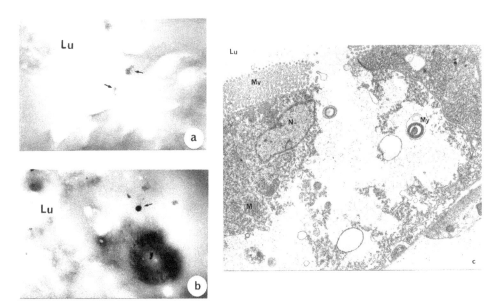

Fig. 6. Metal containing granules in the luminal tube (Lu) of a benthic copepod.
(a) Occurrence of Cu, P, S and Ag in granules (arrows). x ·7 200. (b) Occurrence of Fe, Cu,
Zn, P, S and Ca in a granule (arrow). x ·29 000. (c) Ultrastructure of a digestive cell extruding
its contents into the lumen. Note the presence of a spherocristal, a lysosome which
membrane is electron-dense and another structure with myelin (My). M, mitochondria, Mv,
microvilli, N, nucleus. x ·7 000 (after Barka, 2007).

Once in the gut, the reabsorption of the ions after the granule chemical and enzymatic
dissolution may also occur, as suggested by Becker et al. (1974). Nott and Nicolaidou (1993),
fed a carnivorous gastropod (*Nassarius reticulatus*) with another gastropod (*Littorina littorea*)
hepatopancreas which contained intracellular phosphate granules. These granules passed
through the predator gut. X-Ray microanalysis revealed that granules in the predator faecal
pellets retained about 50% of the original zinc and 33% of the original manganese and showed
that a metal bioreduction occurred along the molluscan food chain suggesting, however, that
part of the metals were bioavailable for the predator. X-ray microanalysis revealed also that, in
phosphate granules, an increase in the quantity of metal is associated with a reduction in the
magnesium/calcium ratio. Metals displace magnesium from the phosphate granule to the
carbonate granule (Nott & Nicolaidou, 1989b; Schönborn et al., 2001).

The ability of granules to dissolve or not in the predator lumen may have a consequence not
only on the trophic transfer of metals but also on the subsequent handling of toxic metals in
predators.

5. Conclusion

Various examples of trace metal bioaccumulation structures, mostly among marine
invertebrates, were illustrated and discussed in this chapter. They revealed the potential of

X-Ray analysis in understanding cellular mechanisms underneath metal bioaccumulation, granule composition, origin, growth and trophic transfer as well as metal detoxification adaptive strategies. For its accuracy and precision, X-Ray microanalysis is a powerful technique which allows to resolve several questions about metal handling. In fact, the way marine animals cope with the presence of metals in their surrounding is still open to investigation. Hence, and in order to enable the monitoring of metals in the environment, granule microanalysis may be proposed as a new approach (Dimitriadis & Papadaki, 2004).

6. Acknowledgments

This chapter has been written in memory of Christiane Ballan-Dufrançais, who left us too early, and to whom I am indebted. I would like to thank Anne-Yvonne Jeantet, Lydia Massot, Anny Anglo and Patricia Beaunier for their technical help and scientific advices.

7. References

Ahsanullah, M., Williams, A.R. (1991). Sublethal effects and bioaccumulation of cadmium, chromium, copper and zinc in the marine amphipod *Allorchestes compressa*. *Marine Biology*, Vol. 108, No. 1, pp (59-65), ISSN 0025-3162

Al-Mohanna, S.Y., Nott, J.A. (1987). R-Cells and the digestive cycle in *Penaeus semisulcatus* (Crustacea : Decapoda). *Marine Biology*, Vol. 95, pp (129-137), ISSN 0025-3162

Amiard, J.C., Amiard-Triquet, C., Berthet, B., Metayer, C. (1987). Comparative study of the patterns of bioaccumulation of essential (Cu, Zn) and non-essential (Cd, Pb) trace metals in various estuarine and coastal organisms. *Journal of Experimental Marine Biology and Ecology*, Vol. 106, pp (73-89), ISSN 0022-0981

Amiard, JC, Amiard-Triquet, C., Barka, S., Pellerin, J., Rainbow, P.S. (2006). Metallothioneins in aquatic invertebrates : Their role in metal detoxification and their use as biomarkers. *Aquatic Toxicology*, Vol. 76, pp (160-202), ISSN 0166-445X

Amiard-Triquet, C., Jeantet, A.Y., Berthet, B. (1993). Metal transfer in marine food chains : bioaccumulation and toxicity. *Acta Biologica Hungarica*, Vol. 44, No. 4, pp (387-409), ISSN 0236-5383

Ballan-Dufrançais, C. (1975). Bioaccumulation minérale , purique et flavinique chez les insectes. Méthodes d'étude-Importance physiologique. *Thèse d'état*, université Pierre-et-Marie-Curie, 172p.

Ballan-Dufrançais, C. (2002). Localization of metals in cells of Pterygote insects. *Microscopy Research and Techniques*, Vol. 56, pp (82-98), ISSN 1059-910X

Ballan-Dufrançais, C. ; Jeantet, A.Y., Halpern, S. (1982). Localisation intracellulaire par microanalyse X de métaux et métalloïdes dans la glande digestive d'un mollusque bivalve (*Pecten maximus*). Implication des processus de digestion. *Comptes-Rendus Hebdomadaires des Séances de l'Académie des Sciences de Paris*, Vol. 294, pp (673-678), ISSN 0567-655X

Barka S. (2000) - Processus de détoxication et localisation tissulaire des métaux traces (cuivre, zinc, nickel, cadmium, argent et mercure) chez un Crustacé marin (Copépode harpacticoïde) *Tigriopus brevicornis*. Etude du biomarqueur « protéines type métallothionéines », de la bioaccumulation des métaux et des conséquences sur le transfert trophique. *Thèse de Doctorat (PhD) de l'Université Pierre et Marie Curie*, p. 204 + Boards

Barka, S. (2007). Insoluble detoxification of trace metals (copper, zinc, nickel, cadmium, silver and mercury) in a marine crustacean *Tigriopus brevicornis* (Müller). *Ecotoxicology*, Vol. 16, pp (491–502), ISSN 0963-9292

Barka, S., Pavillon J.-F., Amiard-Triquet, C. (2010). Metal distribution in *Tigriopus brevicornis* (Crustacea, Copepoda) of copper, zinc, nickel, cadmium, silver and mercury and assessment of subsequent transfer in the food web. *Environmental Toxicology*, Vol. 25, pp (350-360), ISSN 1520-4081

Becker, G.L., Chen, C.H., Greenawalt, J.W., Lehninger, A.L. (1974). Calcium phosphate granules in the hepatopancreas of the blue crab *Callinectes sapidus*. *The Journal of Cell Biology*, Vol. 61, pp (316-326), ISSN 0021-9525

Bernard, F.J., Lane, C.E. (1961). Absorption and excretion of copper ion during settlement and metamorphosis of the barnacle *Balanus amphitrite niveus*. *Biological Bulletin*, Vol. 121, pp (438-488), ISSN 0006-3185

Borgmann, U., Norwood, W.P., Clarcke, C. (1993). Accumulation, regulation and toxicity of copper, zinc, lead and mercury in *Hyatella azteca*. *Hydrobiologia*, Vol. 259, pp (79-89), ISSN 0018-8158

Börjesson, J., Mattsson, S. (2004). New applications. X-Ray fluorescence analysis in medical sciences. In: *X-Ray Spectrometry: Recent Technological Advances*, Tsuji, K., Injuk, J., Van Grieken, R., pp (487-515), John Wiley & Sons, Ltd, ISBN 0-471-48640-X, Chichester

Bouquegneau, J.M., Martoja, M. (1982). Copper content and its degree of complexation in four marine gastropods. Data concerning cadmium and zinc. *Oceanologica Acta*, Vol. 5, No 2, pp (219-231), ISSN 0399-1784

Brown, B.E. (1982). The form and function of metal-containing 'granules' in invertebrate tissues. *Biological Reviews*, Vol. 57, pp (621-667), ISSN 1464-7931

Bruland, K.W. (1983). Trace elements in seawater. In: *Chemical Oceanography 8*, Riley, J.P., Chester, R., pp (157-220), Academic Press, ISBN 0–12-588608-X, London

Bryan, G. W., Langston, W. J. (1992). Bioavailability, accumulation and effects of heavy metals in sediments with special reference to United Kingdom estuaries: a review. *Environmental Pollution*, Vol. 76, No. 2, pp (89-131), ISSN 0269-7491

Bryan, G.W. (1979). Bioaccumulation of marine pollutants. *Philosophical Transactions of the Royal Society of London*, Vol. B286, pp (483-505), ISSN 0080-4622

Bryan, G.W., Gibbs, P.E. (1980). Metals in nereid polychaetes: the contribution of metals in the jaws to the total body burden. *Journal of the Marine Biology Association of the United Kingdom*, Vol. 60, pp (641-654), ISSN 0025-3154

Bury, N.R., Walker, P.A., Clover, C.N., (2003). Nutritive metal uptake in teleost fish. *Journal of Experimental Biology*, Vol. 206, pp (11-23), ISSN 0022-0949

Bustamante, P. (1998). Bioaccumulation des éléments traces chez les mollusques céphalopodes et bivalves pectinidés. Implication de leur biodisponibilité pour le transfert vers les prédateurs. *Thèse de doctorat*, université de La Rochelle, 296p.

Campbell, P.G.C., Tessier, A. (1996). Ecotoxicology of metals in the aquatic environment : Geochemical aspects. In: *Ecotoxicology: A hierarchical treatment*, Newman, M.C., Jagoe, C.H., Lewis Publishers, , pp (11-58), ISBN 1566701279, Boca Raton, Florida

Carmichael, N.G., Squibb, K.S., Fowler, B.A. (1979). Metals in the molluscan kidney : a comparison of two closely related bivalve species (*Argopecten*), using X-ray microanalysis and atomic absorption spectroscopy. *Journal of the Fisheries Research Board of Canada*, Vol. 36, pp (1149-1155), ISSN 0015-296X

Chavez-Crooker, P., Garrido, N. Pozo, P., Ahearn, G.A., (2003). Copper transport by lobster (*Homarus americanus*) hepatopancreatic lysosomes. *Comparative Biochemistry and Physiology*, Vol. C 135, pp (107-118), ISSN 1532-0456

Chen J.C., Liu, P.C. (1987). Accumulation of heavy metals in the nauplii of *Artemia salina*. *Journal of the World Aquaculture Society*, Vol. 18, No. 2, pp (84-93), ISSN 1749-7345

Cheung, V.W.K., Marshall, A.T. 1973. Studies on water and ion transport in homopteran insects: ultrastructure and cytochemistry of the cicadoid and cercopoid midgut. *Tissue and Cell*, Vol. 5, pp (651-669), ISSN 0040-8166

Chou, C.L., Paon, L., Moffatt, J., Zwicker, B. (1998). Concentrations of metals in the American lobster (*Homarus americanus*) and sediments from harbours of the eastern and southern shores and the Annapolis Basin of Nova Scotia, Canada *Canadian Technical Report of Fisheries and Aquatic Sciences*, Vol. 2254, pp (78-89), ISSN 0706-6457

Clason, B., Dusquene, M., Liess, M., Schulz, R., Zauke, G.P. (2003). Bioaccumulation of trace metals in the antarctic amphipod *Paramoera walkeri* (Stebbing, 1906): comparison of two-compartment and hyperbolic toxicokinetic models. *Aquatic Toxicology*, Vol. 65, pp (117-140), ISSN 0166-445X

Corrêa J.D.Jr., Farina, M., Allodi, S. (2002). Cytoarchitectural features of *Ucides cordatus* (Crustacea Decapoda) hepatopancreas: structure and elemental composition of electron-dense granules *Tissue and Cell*, Vol 34, No. 5, (October 2002), pp (315-325), ISSN 0040-8166

Cosson, R.P., Amiard-Triquet, C., Amiard, J.C. (1991). Metallothioneins and detoxification. Is the use of detoxification protein for MTs a language abuse?. *Water Air Soil Pollution*, Vol. 57-58, pp (555-567), ISSN 0049-6979

De Nicola, M., Cardellichio, N., Gambardella, C., Guarino, S.M., Marra, C. (1993). Effects of Cadmium on survival, bioaccumulation, histopathology and PGM polymorphism in the marine isopod *Idothea baltica*, In: *Ecotoxicology of metals in invertebrates,* Dallinger, R., Rainbow, P.S., pp (103-116), SETAC special publication, Lewis Publishers, ISBN 0-87371-734-I, Boca Raton, Florida

Defaye, D., Suck J., Dussart, B. (1985). The alimentary canal of a freshwater Copepoda, *Macrocyclops albidus* and some other Cyclopoida. *Acta Zoologica*, Vol. 66, No. 2, pp (119-129), ISSN 1463-6395

Depledge, M.H., Bjerregaard, P. (1989). Haemolymph protein composition and copper levels in decapods crustaceans. *Helgolander Wissenschaftliche Meeresuntersuchungen*, Vol. 43, pp (207-223), ISSN 0017-9957

Desouky, M.A. (2006). Tissue distribution and subcellular localization of trace metals in the pond snail *Lymnaea stagnalis* with special reference to the role of lysosomal granules in metal sequestration *Aquatic Toxicology*, Vol. 77, No. 2, (May 2006), pp (143-152), ISSN 0166-445X

Dimitriadis, V. K., Papadaki, M. (2004). Field application of autometallography and X-ray microanalysis using the digestive gland of the common mussel. *Ecotoxicology and Environmental Safety*, Vol. 59, No. 1, (September 2004), pp (31-37), ISSN 0147-6513

Durfort, M. (1981). Mineral concretions in the intestinal epithelium of *Cyclops strenuus* Fish (Crustacea: Copepoda). Ultrastructural study. *Butlletit del Institut Catalan de Historia Natural*, Vol. 47, No. 4, pp (93-103), ISSN 1133-6889

Fan, W., Cui, M., Liu, H., Wang, C., Shi, Z., Tan, C., Yang, X. (2011). Nano-TiO2 enhances the toxicity of copper in natural water to Daphnia magna. *Environmental Pollution*, Vol.159, pp (729-734), ISSN 0269-7491

Fowler, B.A. (1987). Intracellular compartmentation of metals in aqautic organisms: Relatioships to mechanisms of cell injury. *Environmental Health Perspectives*, Vol. 71, pp (121-135), ISSN 0091-6765

George, N.G. (1993). X-ray absorption spectroscopy of light elements in biological systems, *Current Opinion in Structural Biology*, Vol. 3, pp (780-784), ISSN 0959-440X

George, S.G. (1982). Subcellular accumulation and detoxication of metals in aquatic organisms. In: *Physiological Mechanisms of Marine Pollutant Toxicity*, Vernberg, W.B. Calabrese, A., Thruberg, F.P., Vernberg, F.J., pp (3-52), Academic Press, ISBN 0-87371-734, New York

George, S.G. (1983a). Heavy metal detoxication in the mussel *Mytilus edulis* - Composition of Cd-containing kidney granules (tertiary lysosomes). *Comparative Biochemistry and Physiology*, Vol. 76, No. 1C, pp (53-57), ISSN 1532-0456

George, S.G. (1983b). Heavy metal detoxication in *Mytilus* kidney – an in vitro study of Cd and Zn-binding to isolated tertiary lysosomes. *Comparative Biochemistry and Physiology*, Vol. 76, No. 1C, pp (59-65), ISSN 1532-0456

Gibbs,. P.E., Bryan, G.W. (1980). Copper-The major inorganic component of glycerid polychaete jaws. *Journal of the Marine Biology Association of the United Kingdom*, Vol. 60, pp (205-214), ISSN 0025-3154

Guary, J.C., Négrel, R. (1981). Calcium phosphate granules : A trap for transuranics and iron in crab hepatopancreas. *Comparative Biochemistry and Physiology*, Vol. 68A, pp (423-427), ISSN 1095-6433

Hogstrand, C., Wood, C.M., (1998). Toward a better understanding of the bioavailability, physiology, and toxicity of silver in fish: implications for water quality criteria. *Environmental Toxicology and Chemistry*, Vol. 17, pp (547–561), ISSN 1552-8618

Hopkin,, S.P., Nott, J.A. (1979). Some observations on concentrically structured intracellular granules in the hepatopancreas of the shore crab *Carcinus maenas* (L.) with special reference to the B-Cells in the hepatopancreas. *Journal of the Marine Biological Association of the United Kingdom*, Vol. 60, pp (891-907), ISSN 0025-3154

Hopkin, S.P., Nott, J.A. (1980). Studies on the digestive cycle of the shore crab *Carcinus maenas* (L.). *Journal of the Marine Biological Association of the United Kingdom*, Vol. 59, pp (867-877), ISSN 0025-3154

Hopkin, S.P. (Ed.). (1989). *Ecophysiology of metals in terrestrial invertebrates*. Elsevier Applied Sciences, ISBN 1-85166-312-6, London

Isheii, T., Ikuta, K., Hara, M., Ishikawa, M., Koyanagi, T. (1986). High accumulation of elements in the kidney of the marine bivalve *Cyclosunetta menstrualis*. *Bulletin of the Japanese Society of Scientific Fisheries*, Vol. 52, pp (147-154), ISSN 0021-5392

Jacob, D.E., Wirth, R., Soldati, A.L., Wehrmeister, U., Schreiber, A. (2011). Amorphous calcium carbonate in the shells of adult *Unionoida*. *Journal of Structural Biology*, Vol. 173, No. 2, (February 2011), pp (241-249), ISSN 1047-8477

Jeantet, A.Y., Ballan-Dufrançais, C., Anglo, A. (1997). Pollution par les métaux et atteintes cytologiques chez les bivalves marins. In: *Biomarqueurs en écotoxicologie. Aspects fondamentaux*, Lagadic, L., Caquet, T., Amiard, J.C., Ramade, F., pp (315-353), ISBN 2225830533, Masson, Paris,

Jones, D.A., Babbage, P.C., King, P.E. (1969). Studies on the digestion and the fine structure of digestive caeca in *Eurydice pulchra* (Crustacea : Isopoda). *Marine Biology*, Vol. 2, pp (311-320), ISSN 0025-3162

Kahle, J., Zauke G.P. (2002a). Bioaccumulation of trace metals in the copepod *Calanoides acutus* from the Weddell Sea (Antarctica): comparison of two-compartment and hyperbolic toxicokinetic models. *The Science of the Total Environment*, Vol. 295, pp (1-16), ISSN 0048-9697

Kahle, J., Zauke, G.-P. (2002b). Bioaccumulation of trace metals in the copepod *Calanoides acutus* from the Weddell Sea (Antarctica): Comparison of two-compartment and hyperbolic toxicokinetic models. *Aquatic Toxicology*, Vol. 59, pp (115-135), ISSN 0166-445X

Khan, F.R., Bury, N.R., Hogstrand, C. (2010). Cadmium bound to metal rich granules and exoskeleton from *Gammarus pulex* causes increased gut lipid peroxidation in zebrafish following single dietary exposure. *Aquatic Toxicology*, Vol. 96, No. 2, (31 January 2010), pp (124-129), ISSN 0166-445X

Kramer, J.R., Benoit, G., Bowles, K.C., Di Toro, D.M., Herrin, R.T., Luther III, G.W., Manolopoulos, H., Robillard, K.A., Shafer, M.M., Shaw, J.R. (2002). . In: *Environmental chemistry of silver, Silver in the Environment: Transport, Fate and Effects*, Andren, A.W., Bober, T.W. (Eds.), pp (1-25), Setac Press, ISBN 0-936287-05-5, Pensacola, FL, USA

Krueger, R.A., Broce, A.B., Hopkins, T.L. (1987). Dissolution of granules in the Malpighian tubules of *Musca autumnalis* DeGeer, during mineralization of the puparium. *Journal of Insect Physiology*, Vol. 33, No. 4, pp (255-263), ISSN 0022-1910

Loret, S.M., Devos, P.E. (1995). Corrective note about R*cells of the digestive gland of the shore crab *Carcinus maenas*. *Cell Tissue Research*, Vol. 290, pp (401-405), ISSN 0302-766X

Lukyanova, O.N., Belcheva, N.N., Chelomin, V.P. (1993). Cadmium bioaccumulation in the scallop *Mizuhopecten yessoensis* from an unpolluted environment. In: *Ecotoxicology of metals in invertebrates*, Dallinger, R., Rainbow, P.S., pp (103-116), SETAC special publication, pp (26-35), Lewis Publishers, ISBN 0-87371-734-I, Boca Raton, Florida

Maranhao, P., Marques, J.C., Madeira, V.M.C. (1999). Zinc and cadmium concentrations in soft tissues of the red swamp crayfish *Procambarus clarkii* (Girard 1852) after exposure to zinc and cadmium. *Environmental Toxicology and Chemistry*, Vol. 18, No. 8, pp (1769-1771), ISSN 1552-8618

Marigomez, J.A., Cajaraville, M.P., Angulo, E. (1990). Cellular cadmium distribution in the common winkle *Littorina littorea* (L.) determined by X-ray microprobe analysis and histochemistry. *Histochemistry*, Vol. 94, pp (191-199), ISSN 0301-5564

Marigomez, J.A., Soto, M., Carajaville, M.P., Angulo, E., Giamberini, L. (2002). Cellular and subcellular distribution of metals in molluscs, *Microscopy Research and Techniques*, Vol. 56, pp (358-392), ISSN 1059-910X

Contribution of X-Ray Spectroscopy to Marine Ecotoxicology: Trace Metal Bioaccumulation and Detoxification
in Marine Invertebrates

45

Marsden, I.D., Rainbow, P.S. (2004). Does the accumulation of trace metals in crustaceans affect their ecology—the amphipod example? *Journal of Experimental Marine Biology and Ecology*, Vol.300, No. 1-2, pp (373-408), ISSN 0022-0981

Marsh, M.E., Sass, R.L. (1985). Distribution and characterization of mineral-binding phosphoprotein particles in Bivalvia. *Journal of Experimental Zoology*, *Vol.* 234, pp (237-242), ISSN 0022-104X

Martoja, M., Bouquegneau, J.M. , Truchet, M. , Martoja, B. (1985). Recherche de l'argent chez quelques mollusques marins, dulcicoles et terrestres. Formes chimiques et localisation histologiques. *Vie et Milieu*, Vol. 35, No. 1, pp (1-13), ISSN 0506-8924

Martoja, M., Tue, V.T., Elkaïm, B. (1980). Bioaccumulation du cuivre chez *Littorina littorea* (L.) (Gastéropode, Prosobranche). Signification physiologique et écologique. *Journal of Experimental Marine Biology and Ecology*, Vol. 43, pp (251-270), ISSN 0022-0981

Martoja, M., Ballan-Dufrançais, C., Jeantet, A.Y., Truchet, M., Coulon, J. (1988). Influence de la composition chimique de l'environnement sur le bivalve *Abra alba*. Etude comparative d'animaux récoltés dans des milieux naturels et d'animaux contaminés expérimentalement par un effluent industriel. *Annales de l'Institut Océanographique*, Vol.64, No. 1, pp (1-24), ISSN 0078-9682

Masala, O., McInnes, E.J.L., O'Brien, P. (2002). Modelling the formation of granules: the influence of manganese ions on calcium pyrophosphate precipitates. *Inorganica Chimica Acta*, Vol. 339, pp (366-372), ISSN 0020-1693

Masala, O., O'Brien, P., Rainbow, P.S., (2004). Analysis of metal-containing granules in the barnacle *Tetraclita squamosa*. *Journal of Inorganic Biochemistry*, Vol. 98, pp (1095-1102), ISSN 0162-0134

Mason, A.Z., Simkiss, K., Ryan, K. (1984). Ultrastructural localization of metals in specimens in *Littorina littorea* (L.) from polluted and non-polluted sites. *Journal of the Marine Biological Association of the United Kingdom*, Vol. 64, pp (699-720), ISSN 0025-3154

Mason, A.Z., Nott, J.A. (1981). The role of intracellular biomineralized granules in the regulation and detoxification of metals in gastropods with special reference ti the marine prosobranch *Littorina littorea*. *Aquatic Toxicology*, Vol. 1, pp (239-256), ISSN 0166-445X

Mason, A.Z., Jenkins, K.D. (1995). Metal detoxification in aquatic organisms. In: *Metal speciation and bioavailability in aquatic systems*, Tessier A., Turner, D.R., John Wiley & Sons Ltd, pp (479-608), ISBN 0-471-95830-1, London,

Mason, A.Z., Simkiss, K. (1982). Sites of mineral deposition in metal accumulating cells. *Experimental Cell Research*, Vol. 139, pp (383-391), ISSN 0014-4827

Moore, P.G. (1979). Crystalline structure in the gut caeca of the amphipod *Stegocephaloides christaniensis* Boeck *Journal of Experimental Marine Biology and Ecology*, Vol. 39, pp (223-229), ISSN 0022-0981

Moore, P.G., Rainbow, P.S. (1992). Aspects of the biology of iron, copper and other metals in relation to feeding in *Andaniexis abyssi*, with notes on *Andaniopsis nordlandica* and *Stegocephalus inflatus* (Amphipoda: Stegocephalidae), from Norwegian waters. *Sarsia*, Vol. 76, No. 4, pp (215-225), ISSN 0036-4827

Morillo, J., Usero, J., Bakouri, H.E. (2008). Biomonitoring of heavy metals in the coastal waters of two industrialised bays in southern Spain using the barnacle Balanus amphitrite. *Chemical Speciation and Bioavailability*, Vol.20, No. 4, pp (227-237), ISSN 0954-2299

Nassiri, Y., Rainbow, P.S., Amiard-triquet, C., Rainglet, F., Smith, B.D. (2000). Trace metal detoxification in the ventral caeca of *Orchestia gammarellus* (Crustacea: Amphipoda). *Marine Biology*, Vol. 136, pp (477-484), ISSN 0025-3162

Ni, I.H., Wang, W.X., Tam, Y.K. (2000). Transfer of Cd, Cr and Zn from zooplankton prey to mudskipper *Periophthalmus cantonensis* and glassy *Ambassis urotaenia* fishes. *Marine Ecology Progress Series*, Vol. 194, pp (203-210), ISSN 0171-8630

Nott, J.A. (1991). Cytology of pollutant metals in marine invertebrates: A review of microanalytical applications. *Scanning Microscopy*, Vol. 5, pp (191-230), ISSN 0891-7035

Nott, J.A., Nicolaidou, A. (1989a). The cytology of heavy metal accumulation in the digestive glands of three marine gastropods. *Proceedings of the Royal Society of London*, Vol. 234B, pp (463-470), ISSN 0962-8452

Nott, J.A., Nicolaidou, A. (1989b). Metals in gastropods — metabolism and bioreduction *Marine Environmental Research*, Vol. 28, No. 1-4, pp (201-205), ISSN 0141-1136

Nott, J.A., Nicolaidou, A. (1990). Transfer of metal detoxification along marine food chains. *Journal of Marine Biological Association of the United Kingdom*, Vol. 70, pp (905-912), ISSN 0025-315

Nott, J.A., Nicolaidou, A. (1993). Bioreduction of zinc and manganese along a molluscan food chain. *Comparative Biochemistry and Physiology Part A: Physiology*, Vol. 104, No. 2, (February 1993), pp (235-238), ISSN 1095-6433

Pequegnat, J.E., Fowler, S.W., Small, L.F. (1969). Estimates of the zinc requirements of marine organisms. *Journal of the Fisheries Research Board of Canada*, Vol.26, pp (145-150), ISSN 0015-296X

Phillips, D.J.H., Rainbow, P.S. (1988). Barnacles and mussels as biomonitors of trace elements: a comparative study, *Marine Ecology Progress Series*, Vol.49, pp (83-93), ISSN 0171-8630

Pigino, G., Migliorini, M., Paccagnini, E. Bernini F. (2006). Localisation of heavy metals in the midgut epithelial cells of *Xenillus tegeocranus* (Hermann, 1804) (Acari: Oribatida). *Ecotoxicology and Environmental Safety*, Vol. 64, No. 3, (July 2006), pp (257-263), ISSN 0147-6513

Pohl, C. (1992). Wechselbeziehungen zwischen Spurenmetalkonzentrationen (Cd, Cu, Pb, Zn) im meerwasser und in zooplanktonorganismen (Copepoda) der Arktis und des Atlantiks. *Berichte zur Polarforschung*, Vol. 101, pp (1-198), ISSN 0176-5027

Pullen, J.S.H., Rainbow, P.S. (1991). The composition of pyrophosphate heavy metal detoxification granules in barnacles. *Journal of Experimental Marine Biology and Ecology*, Vol. 150, No. 2, pp (249-266), ISSN 0022-0981

Quintana, C., Bonnet, N., Jeantet, AY., Chemelle, P. (1987). Crystallographic study of the ferritin molecules : new results obtained from the natural crystals *in situ* (mollusk oocyte) and from isolated molecules (horse spleen). *Biology of the Cell*, Vol.59, pp (247-254), ISSN 0248-4900

Raimundo, J., Vale, C., Duarte, R., Moura, I. (2008). Sub-cellular partitioning of Zn, Cu, Cd and Pb in the digestive gland of native *Octopus vulgaris* exposed to different metal concentrations (Portugal). *The Science of The Total Environment*, Vol. 390, No. 2-3, (15 February 2008), pp (410-416), ISSN 0048-9697

Rainbow, P.S. (2007). Trace metal bioaccumulation: Models, metabolic availability and toxicity. *Environment International*, Vol.33, No. 4, pp (576-582), ISSN 0160-4120

Contribution of X-Ray Spectroscopy to Marine Ecotoxicology: Trace Metal Bioaccumulation and Detoxification
in Marine Invertebrates

47

Rainbow, P.S., Smith, B.D. (2010). Trophic transfer of trace metals: Subcellular compartmentalization in bivalve prey and comparative assimilation efficiencies of two invertebrate predators *Journal of Experimental Marine Biology and Ecology*, Vol. 390, No. 2, pp (143-148),   0022-0981

Rainbow, P.S. (1987). Heavy metals in barnacles. In: *Crustacean Issues 5-Barnacle Biology*, Southward, A.J. (Ed.), pp (405-407), ISBN 90-6191-628-3, Rotterdam

Rainbow, P.S. (1988). The significance of trace metal concentration in decapods, *Proceeding of the Symposium of the Zoological Society of London*, London, april 1988

Rainbow, P.S. (1993). The significance of trace metal concentration in marine invertebrates. In: *Ecotoxicology of metals in invertebrates*, Dallinger, R., Rainbow, P.S. (Eds.), pp (3-23), SETAC special publication, Lewis Publishers, ISBN 0-87371-734-I, Boca Raton, Florida

Rainbow, P.S. (1997). Trace metal accumulation in marine invertebrates : Marine biology or marine chemistry? *Journal of Marine Biology Association of the United Kingdom*, Vol. 77, pp (195-210), ISSN 0025-3154

Rainbow, P.S. (1998). Phylogeny of trace metal accumulation in crustaceans. In: *Metal Metabolism in Aquatic Environments*, Langston, W.J., Bebianno, M., pp (285-319), Chapman and Hall, ISBN 0412803704, London

Rainbow, P.S., Phillips, D.J.H., Depledge, M.H. (1990). The significance of trace metal concentrations in marine invertebrates, a need for laboratory investigation of accumulation strategies. *Marine Pollution Bulletin*, Vol. 21, pp (321-324), ISSN 0025-326X

Rainbow, P.S., White, S.L. (1989). Comparative strategies of heavy metal accumulation by crustaceans : zinc, copper and cadmium in decapod, an amphipod and a barnacle. *Hydrobiologia*, Vol. 74, pp (243-262), ISSN 0018-8158

Rainbow, P.S., (2002). Trace metal concentrations in aquatic invertebrates: why and so what?. *Environmental Pollution*, Vol. 120, pp (497-507), ISSN 0269-7491

Rainbow, P.S., (2006). Trace metal bioaccumulation: model, metabolic availability and toxicity. *Environment International*, Vol. 30, pp (67-78), ISSN 0160-4120

Rainbow, P.S., Moore, P.G., Watson, D. (1989). Talitrid amphipods as biomonitors for copper and zinc, *Estuarine Coastal Shelf Science*, Vol.28, pp (567-582), ISSN 0272-7714

Rainbow, P.S., Kriefman, S., Smith, B.D., Luoma, S.N. (2011) Have the bioavailabilities of trace metals to a suite of biomonitors changed over three decades in SW England estuaries historically affected by mining? *The Science of The Total Environment*, Vol. 409, No. 8, pp (1589-1602), ISSN 0048-9697

Ramade, F. (Ed.) (1992). *Précis d'écotoxicologie*, Masson, ISBN 2-225-82578-5, Paris

Reid, R.G.B., Brand, D.G. (1989). Giant kidneys and metal sequestering nephroliths in the bivalve *Pinna bicolor*, with comparative notes on *Altrina vexillum* (Pinnidae). *Journal of Experimental Marine Biology and Ecology*, Vol. 126, pp (95-117), ISSN 0022-0981

Reinfelder, J.R., Fisher, N.S. (1991). The assimilation of elements ingested by marine copepods. *Science*, Vol. 251, pp (794-796), ISSN 0036-8075

Reinfelder, J.R., Fisher, N.S. (1994). Retention of elements absorbed by juvenile fish (*Menidia menidia, Menidia beryllina*) from zooplankton prey. *Limnology and Oceanography*, Vol. 39, pp (1783-1789), ISSN 0024-3590

Ridout, P.S., Rainbow, P.S., Roe, H.S., Jones, H.R. (1989). Concentrations of V, Cr, Mn, Fe, Ni, Co, Cu, Zn, As, Cd in mesopelagic crustaceans from north east Atlantic Ocean, *Marine Biology*, Vol.100, pp (465-), ISSN 0025-3162

Ritterhoff, J., Zauke, G.P. (1997a). Bioaccumulation of trace metals in Greeland Sea copepod and amphipod collectives on board ship : verification of toxicokinetic model parameters. *Aquatic Toxicology*, Vol. 40, pp (63-78), ISSN 0166-445X

Ritterhoff, J., Zauke, G.P. (1997b). Trace metals in field samples of zooplankton from the Fram Strait and the Greenland Sea. *The Science of The Total Environment*, Vol. 199, pp (255-270), ISSN 0048-9697

Roesijadi, G., Robinson, W.E. (1994). Metal regulation in aquatic animals: Mechanisms of uptake, accumulation and release. In: *Aquatic toxicology: molecular, biochemical and cellular perspectives*, Martins, D.C., Ostrander, G.K., pp (387-420), Lewis Publishers, ISBN 0-87371-545-4, Boca Raton,.

Rokosz, M.J., Vinogradov, S.N. (1982). X-ray fluorescence spectrometric determination of the metal content of the extracellular hemoglobin of *Tubifex tubifex*. *Biochimica et Biophysica Acta (BBA) - Protein Structure and Molecular Enzymology*, Vol. 707, No. 2, (5 October 1982), pp (291-293), ISSN 0167-4838

Sandler, A. (1984). Zinc and copper concentrations in benthic invertebrates considered in relation to concentrations in sediments and water in the Bothnian sea (Northen Baltic). *Finnish Marine Research*, Vol. 250, pp (19-32), ISSN 0357-1076

Schofield, R.M.S., Niedbala, J.C. Nesson, M.H., Tao, Y., Shokes, J.E., Scott, R.A., Latimer, M.J. (2009). Br-rich tips of calcified crab claws are less hard but more fracture resistant: A comparison of mineralized and heavy-element biological materials. *Journal of Structural Biology*, Vol. 166, No. 3, (June 2009), pp (272-287), ISSN 1047-8477

Schönborn, C., Bauer, H.D., Röske, I. (2001) Stability of enhanced biological phosphorus removal and composition of polyphosphate granules. *Water Research*, Vol.35, No. 13, pp (3190-3196), ISSN 0043-1354

Simkiss, K. (1976). Intracellular and extracellular routes of biomineralization. In: *Calcium in biological systems*, Symposia of the Society for experimental Biology 30, p (423-444), University Press, ISBN 0521212367, Cambridge

Simkiss, K. (1981). Cellular discrimination processes in metal accumulating cells. *Journal of Experimental Biology*, Vol. 94, pp (317-), ISSN 0022-0949

Simkiss, K., Mason, A.Z. (1983). Metal ions: Metabolic and toxic effects. In: *The Mollusca Vol.2*, Wilbur, K.M., pp (101), Academic Press, New York

Simkiss, K., Taylor, M.G. (1989). Metal fluxes across the membranes of aquatic organisms. *CRC Critical Reviews in Aquatic Sciences*, Vol. 1, pp (173-), ISSN 0891-4117

Simkiss, K., Taylor, M.G. (1995). Transport of metals across membranes. In: *Metal speciation and bioavailability in aquatic systems*, Tessier A., Turner, D.R., John Wiley & Sons Ltd, pp (1-44), ISBN 0-471-95830-1, London

Simkiss, K., Wilbur, K.M., (1989). Crustacea—The dynamics of epithelial movements. In: *Biomineralization: Cell Biology and Mineral Deposition*, Simkiss, K., Wilbur, K.M., pp. (205–229), Academic Press, ISBN 978-0-12-643830-7 , San Diego

Simmons, J., Simkiss, K., Taylor, M.G., Jarvis, K.E., (1996). Crab biominerals as environmental monitors. *Bulletin of Institute of Ocean*, Vol. 14, pp (225-231)

Simon, O., Floriani, M., Cavalie, I., Camilleri, V., Adam, C., Gilbin, R., Garnier-Laplace, J. (2011). Internal distribution of uranium and associated genotoxic damages in the chronically exposed bivalve *Corbicula fluminea*. *Journal of Environmental Radioactivity*, Vol. 102, No. 8, (August 2011), pp (766-773), ISSN 0265-931X

Stegeman, J.J., Brouwer, M., Di Giulio, R.T., Förlin, L., Fowler, B.A., Sanders, B.M., Van Veld, P.A. (1992). Molecular responses to environmental contamination: Enzyme and protein systems as indicators of chemical exposure and effect. In: *Biomarkers, Biochemical, Physiological and Histological Markers of Anthropogenic Stress*, Huggett, R.J., Kimerle, R.A., Mehrle, P.M. Jr, Bergman, H.L. pp (235-355),. Lewis Publishers, ISBN 087371-505-5, Boca Raton Florida

Sullivan, P.A., Robinson, W.E., Morse, M.P. (1988). Isolation and characterization of granules from the kidney of the bivalve *Mercenaria mercenaria*. *Marine biology*, Vol. 99, pp(359-367), ISSN 0025-3162

Taylor, M.G., Simkiss, K., Greaves, G.N., Haries, J. (1988). Corrosion of intracellular granules and cell death. *Proceedings of the Royal Society of London*, Vol. 234B, pp(463-476), ISSN 0962-8452

Tupper, C., Pitman, A., Cragg, S. (2000). Copper accumulation in the digestive caecae of *Limnoria quadripunstata* Holthius (Isopoda: Crustacea) tunnelling CCA-treated wood in laboratory cultures. *Holzforschung*, Vol. 54, No. 6, pp (570-576), ISSN 0018-3830

Uma, D.V., Prabhakara, R.Y. (1989). Zinc accumulation in fiddler crabs, *Uca annulipes* Latreille and *Uca triangulis* (Milne Edwards). *Ecotoxicology and Environmental Safety*, Vol. 18, pp (129-140), ISSN 0147-6513

Uthi, J.F., Chou, C.L. (1987). Cadmium in sea scallop (*Placopecten magellanicus*) tissues from clean and contaminated areas. *Canadian Journal of Fisheries and Aquatic Sciences*, Vol.44, pp (91-98), ISSN 0706-652

Van Cappellen, E. (2004) Energie Dispersive X-Ray Microanalysis in Scaning and conventional transmission electronic microscopy. In: *X-Ray Spectrometry: Recent Technological Advances*, Tsuji, K., Injuk, J., Van Grieken, R., pp (387-391), John Wiley & Sons, Ltd, ISBN 0-471-48640-X, Chichester

Vesk, P.A., Byrne, M. (1999). Metal levels in tissue granules of the freshwater bivalve *Hyridella depressa* (Unionida) for biomonitoring: the importance of cryopreparation. *The Science of The Total Environment*, Vol. 225, No. 3, (January 1999), pp (219-229), ISSN 0048-9697

Viarengo, A., Moore, M.N., Mancinelli, P.M., Zanicchi, G., Pipe, R.K. (1987). Detoxification of copper in the cells of the digestive gland of mussels: the role of lysosomes and thioneins. *The Science of the Total Environment*,Vol. 44, pp(135-145), ISSN 0048-9697

Viarengo, A., Nott, J.A. (1993). Mechanisms of heavy metal cation homeostasis in marine invertebrates. *Comparative Biochemistry and Physiology*, Vol. 104C, pp (355 372), ISSN 1532-0456

Vijayram, K., Geraldine, P. (1996). Regulation of essential heavy metals (Cu, Cr, and Zn) by the freshwater prawn *Macrobrachium malcolmsonii* (Milne Edwards). *Bulletin of Environmental Contamination and Toxicology*, Vol. 56, No. 2, pp (335-342), ISSN 0007-4861

Vogt, G., Quinitio, E.T. (1994). Accumulation and excretion of metal granules in the prawn *Penaeus monodon,* exposed to water-borne copper, lead, iron and calcium. *Aquatic Toxicology*, Vol. 28, pp (223-241), ISSN 0166-445X

Walker, G. (1977). "Copper" granules in the barnacle *Balanus balanoides*. *Marine Biology*, vol. 39, pp (343-349), ISSN 0025-3162

Wallace, W.G., Lopez, G.R. (1997). Bioavailability of biologically sequesters cadmium and the implications of metal detoxification. *Marine Ecology Progress Series*, Vol. 147, pp (149-157), ISSN 0171-8630

Wallace, W.G., Lopez, G.R., Levinton, J.S. (1998). Cadmium resistance in an oligochaete and its effects on cadmium trophic transfer to an omnivorous shrimp. *Marine Ecology Progress Series*, Vol. 172, pp (225-237), ISSN 0171-8630

Wang, W.X., Rainbow, P.S. (2008) Comparative approaches to understand metal bioaccumulation in aquatic animals *Comparative Biochemistry and Physiology Part C: Toxicology & Pharmacology*, Vol. 148, No. 4, pp (315-323), ISSN 1532-0456

Wang, W.X., Rainbow, P.S. (2000). Dietary uptake of Cd, Cr and Zn in the barnacle *Balanus trigonus*: influence of diet composition. *Marine Ecology Progress Series*, Vol. 204, pp (159-168), ISSN 0171-8630

Weeks, J.M. (1992). Copper-rich granules in the ventral caeca of talitrid amphipods (Crustacea; Amphipoda: Talitridae). *Ophelia*, Vol. 36, No. 2, pp (119-133), ISSN 0078-5326

White, S.L., Rainbow, P.S. (1984). Regulation of zinc concentration of *Palaemon elegans* (Crustacea: Decapoda): Zinc flux and effects of temperature, zinc concentration and moulting. *Marine Ecology Progress Series*, Vol. 16, pp (135-147), ISSN 0171-8630

White, S.L., Rainbow, P.S. (1985). On the metabolic requirements for copper and zinc in molluscs and crustaceans. *Marine Environmental Research*, Vol. 16, pp (215-229), ISSN 0141-1136

Zauke, G.P., Krause, M., Weber, A. (1996). Trace metals in mesozooplankton of the north sea : concentrations in different taxa and preliminary results on bioaccumulation in copepod collectives (*Calanus finmarchicus/C. helgolandicus*). *Intenational Revue der Gesamten und Hydrographie. Systematische beihefte*, Vol. 81, pp (141-160), ISSN 0535-4137

Zafiropoulos, D., Grimanis, A.P. (1977). Trace elements in *Acartia clausi* from Elefis Bay of the upper Saronikos Gulf, Greece. *Marine Pollution Bulletin*, Vol. 8, pp (79-81), ISSN 0025-326X

Zauke, G.P., Petri, G. (1993). Metal concentration in Antarctic Crustacea: the problem of background levels. In: *Ecotoxicology of metals in invertebrates*, Dallinger, R., Rainbow, P.S., pp (73-101), SETAC special publication, Lewis Publishers, ISBN 0-87371-734-I, Boca Raton, Florida

3

Patulin Analysis:
Sample Preparation Methodologies
and Chromatographic Approaches

Sara Pires, João Lopes, Inês Nunes and Elvira Gaspar
*CQFB-REQUIMTE/Departamento de Química/Faculdade
de Ciências e Tecnologia/Universidade Nova de Lisboa
Portugal*

1. Introduction

Patulin is a mycotoxin with carcinogenic, mutagenic and teratogenic potential mainly produced by several species of *Pennicillium, Aspergillus* and *Byssoclamys*. This toxin has been found in fresh food such as fruits and vegetables, but may also be present in commercial apple juices and other food products. Food contamination with this toxin had led, over the years, to intense investigations related with its occurrence, toxicity, and also to develop prevention and detoxification methods from human and animal food chains. Patulin occurrence compelled several regulating entities to establish maximum limits in some food products, and thereupon, the identification and quantification of this mycotoxin demands the development of sensitive, selective and effective analytical methods.

2. Fungi and mycotoxins

Fungus is an organism which used to be traditionally included in the plant family, but nowadays belongs to the Fungi kingdom due to their considerable differences to plants, such as their inability to produce their own food. They are cosmopolitan in distribution, generally unnoticed due to small size. Nevertheless, these organisms have been applied in the food industry, used as sources of pharmaceutical agents for the treatment of infectious and metabolic diseases, and have shown high importance in agriculture due to their ability to establish symbiotic relationships with plants roots.

Fungi obtain their food through organic matter decomposition, creating at that stage an excellent opportunity for their growth in food. Fungal growth may result in production of toxins harmful to human health causing mycotoxicoses (Bennett, 1987).

In a brief chemical description, mycotoxins can be introduced as low-molecular-weight natural products, with great structural diversity, produced as secondary metabolites by fungi (Bennett & Klich, 2003). These fungi possess the ability to infect food, causing intoxication in animals and humans through contamination of crops or foods prepared from them, reason why the term mycotoxin comes from the fusion of the Greek word *mykes* and the Latin *toxicum*, meaning fungus and toxin, respectively. At this point, it is clear that mycotoxins are toxic compounds; but the definition of mycotoxin refers specifically to metabolites toxic to vertebrates in low concentration (Bennett, 1987). Nevertheless, not all toxic compounds produced by fungi can be defined as mycotoxins, and a good example of this is the antibiotic penicillin, produced by *Penicillium* fungi, which is especially toxic to bacteria.

Common observation one can find in fungi kingdom is that mould species produces more than one type of mycotoxin, and the same mycotoxin can be produced by different types of moulds (Robbins et al., 2000, as cited in Ciegler & Bennett, 1980).

2.1 Toxicology and human health

Mycoses are infections caused by fungal growth on a host, and mycotoxicoses are intoxications, which occur as a consequence from different exposures sources such as food intake, respiratory and dermal contacts. Mycotoxicoses are similar to several other types of intoxications and their symptoms are quite dependent on the specific mycotoxin which causes the illness, the extent of exposure, age, gender and health of the individual, and other aspects like genetics and drug interactions. In the worst cases, mycotoxin poisoning can be amplified due to factors like sub nutrition, alcohol abuse and the presence of other diseases (Bennett & Klich, 2003).

Mycotoxicoses syndromes can be categorized as acute or chronic, and can range from rapid death to tumor development. Other less revealing diseases may occur when the mycotoxin interferes with immune system, leaving it susceptible to infectious diseases. The recognition of a mycotoxicoses is a long way to run. To do so, a dose-response relationship is required to recognize correctly the illness and associate it with the mycotoxin which caused it. Therefore, it is imperative to perform epidemiologic studies in the human population. The common way to execute these studies is by analogy, where a controlled animal population is subjected to a mycotoxin and human syndromes are reproduced. Human exposure to mycotoxins can also be determined by environmental or biological monitoring. In environmental monitoring, mycotoxins are measured in food, air, or other samples that may be in contact with the subjects, while in biological monitoring quantitative and qualitative evaluations of residues are made, and adducts and metabolites in tissue fragments, bodily fluids and excreta (Bennet & Klich, 2003, as cited in Hsieh, 1988) are evaluated.

Fungal diseases are considered to be a severe health problem worldwide.

2.2 Food contaminants

Nowadays, the use of botanical products is increasing due to the importance of diets and life style for human beings and, consequently, the quality of food products is fundamental. In developed countries, botanical products are recommended for medicinal and general health-promoting purposes. However, numerous occurrences of natural mycotoxins in botanicals and fruits have been reported, bringing along food spoilage and considerable economic losses.

Despite the development and industrialization of a country, mycotoxins can occur when environmental, social and economic conditions combined with meteorological conditions (humidity, temperature) promote growth of moulds. Therefore, from an ecological point of view, the role of mycotoxins in disease inducement should not be disregarded. For example, the current trade patterns, mycotoxicoses resulting from contaminated food, locally grown or imported, could occur worldwide. And as consequence, it would be wrong to state that mycotoxin exposure only occurs in underdeveloped countries in which the population is malnourished and there is no regards in food handling and storage (Peraica et al., 1999).

The use of preventive techniques for the control of fungal growth in agricultural commodities and to improve methods for food preparation in industrial standards and food spoilage are never successful. For instance, taste, size, shape, texture and appearance are the basic features of evaluation of a fruit, these will dictate the fruit final destination, consumption or processing. In other hand, food products made from fruits are classified according to their quality using indicators of contamination. Specifically in food products, quality can be characterized by the growth of observable fungi, the existence of unpleasant odor and decomposition of the fruit. In the presence of a fungal contamination, a fruit can exhibit a profound change due to production of disintegrative pectinolytic enzymes responsible for the fruit tissues degradation.

As it was mentioned before, food contamination with mycotoxins is dependent of the influence of environmental and biological factors that determine the fungi production. These factors include the composition of the substrate, temperature, humidity, pH, microbial competition and insect damage (Songsermsakul & Razzazi-Fazeli, 2008; Sant'Ana et al., 2008). Contamination occurs during growing, harvesting, transportation, storage and/or processing of food products (Sant'Ana et al., 2008). As an example, *Aspergillus* and *Penicillium* species are usually associated with contamination during storage, whereas *Fusarium* species can produce mycotoxins before or right after harvesting (Abramson et al., 1997).

Contaminated feed for animals may also have deleterious effects on humans through food chain. In fact, the animal derived products like milk, eggs and meat may appear contaminated with chemicals produced by fungi (Shephard, 2008; Krska et al., 2008).

Beyond the devastating effect of agricultural growth of fungi, toxins produced by them have harmful effects on human health, including carcinogenicity, teratogenicity and growth retardation (Shephard, 2008). Aflatoxins, citrinin, fumonisin (Figure 1), ochratoxin, patulin, trichothecenes and zearalenone are among the mycotoxins that have received more attention in recent years due to their frequent occurrence and their effects on human health (Bennett & Klich, 2003).

2.3 Patulin

Patulin (Figure 2) was initially classified as broad-spectrum antifungal antibiotic. Later, it was found to inhibit more than seventy five different species of bacteria. Further investigations also revealed patulin's violent toxicity to animals and plants (Ciegler et al., 1971).

Patulin (PAT), IUPAC name 4-hydroxy-4H-furo[3,2-c]pyran-2(6H)-one, is characterized by being a hemiacetal lactone, with empirical formula $C_7H_6O_4$, molecular weight 154.12 g/mol, with an appearance of white powder and a melting point of 110°C. Patulin presents a very intense maximum UV absorption at 276 nm (Ciegler et al., 1971; Nielsen & Smedsgaard, 2003).

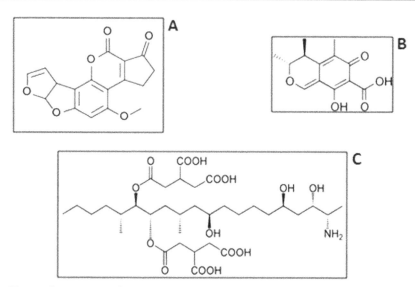

Fig. 1. Chemical structures of some common mycotoxins: aflotoxin B_1 (A), citrinin (B) and fumonisin B_1 (C).

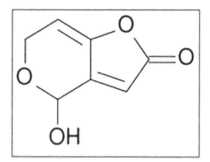

Fig. 2. Patulin chemical structure.

Patulin is an organic compound very soluble in water and in most organic solvents. It is stable in diluted acids and resistant to temperatures at 125°C in the 3.5 - 5.5 pH range (Collin et al., 2008, as cited in Lovett & Peeler, 1973).

2.3.1 Sources and natural occurrence

The main   species of fungi which produce patulin in food are *Aspergillus, Penicillium, Byssochlamys*. *Penicillium expansum* has been identified as the major producer of patulin from the *Penicillium* species (Ciegler et al., 1971, as cited in Shibata et al., 1964) which is responsible for the vast majority of spoiled fruit. Both *Penicillium* and *Aspergillus* have the ability to grow at low temperatures. On the other hand, the fungi of the genus *Byssochlamys* are responsible for patulin production in post-pasteurization stages. This production is due to the fungi ability to survive the heat treatments which are applied to food products (Sant'Ana et al., 2008).

Fungal strains which produce patulin have been isolated over the years from various fruits and vegetables. Although patulin can occur in several fruits, grains and other foods infected by fungi, the main concern is with apples (Sommer et al., 1974, as cited in Brian et al., 1956; Harwig et al., 1973), apple cider (Sands et al., 1976, as cited in Stott &.Bullernan, 1975) and apple juice (Scott et al., 1972) due to their higher consumption. It is also found and isolated from other fruits and vegetables; they are: grapes, pears, apricots (Sommer et al., 1974), cherries, strawberries, nectarines, raspberries, peaches, plums, tomatoes, bananas, almonds, hazelnuts and peanuts (Leggott & Shephard, 2001; Moake et al., 2005, as cited in Harvey et al., 1972; Buchanan et al., 1974; Lovett et al., 1974; Akerstrand et al., 1976; Andersson et al., 1977; Frank et al., 1977; Harwig et al., 1978; Brackett & Marth, 1979a; Jelinek et al., 1989; Jiminez et al., 1991; Prieta et al., 1994; Demirci et al., 2003; Ritieni, 2003).

Studies have been developed in several countries related with the occurrence of patulin; it has been identified in apples from Canada, England, United States, Australia (Sommer et al., 1974), South Africa (Leggott & Shephard, 2001), New Zealand (Moake et al., 2005, as cited in Walker, 1969) and Portugal (Gaspar & Lucena, 2009), and had also been found in apple juices from Canada (Moake et al., 2005, as cited in Scott et al., 1972), United States (Moake et al., 2005, as cited in Ware et al., 1974), Sweden (Moake et al., 2005, as cited in Josefsson & Andersson, 1976), South Africa (Leggott & Shephard, 2001), Turkey (Gokmen & Acar, 1998), Brazil (Moake et al., 2005, as cited in de Sylos & Rodriquez-Amaya, 1999), Austria (Moake et al., 2005, as cited in Steiner et al., 1999a), Italy (Moake et al., 2005, as cited in Ritieni, 2003), Belgium (Moake et al., 2005, as cited in Tangi et al., 2003), and Portugal (Gaspar & Lucena, 2009; Barreira et al, 2010).

2.3.2 Ecotoxicology and legal relevance

In the last decades, attempts have been made to carry out the work on the risk caused by patulin on human health. In the early 1940's, a work reported a metabolic compound derived from a *Penicillium* species, called patulin, which had the potential of being applied in the treatment to the common cold (Medical Research Council, 2004, as cited in Raistrick, 1943), but no evidence was found that patulin would be effective in the treatment of that disease. Due to its toxic evidenced effects, such as nausea, vomiting and gastrointestinal disturbances, patulin did not prove to be an efficient drug.

In the same decade, under the common name clavacin, a study of its antibiotic properties was performed. Preliminary results from this study showed that it was active against Gram-negative and Gram-positive bacteria, but it was also highly toxic to animal organisms (Katzman et al., 1944, as cited in Waksman et al., 1942).

Since then, several *in vitro* and *in vivo* studies have been performed to evaluate the toxicological risk associated with patulin consumption through fresh and processed food products, and other exposure types. In one of these chemical researches, patulin showed a strong affinity for sulfhydryl groups. The compound detains a great ability to form adducts with cysteine, although these adducts are less toxic than the unmodified toxin, respecting acute toxicity, teratogenicity, and mutagenicity studies. Its affinity for sulfhydryl groups explains the inhibition of many enzymes (Ciegler et al., 1976). Although the data on genotoxicity were variable, most assays carried out with mammalian cells were positive, while assays with bacteria were mainly negative. After acute administration and short-term studies, the main signals of toxicity caused by patulin were gastrointestinal hyperemia, distension, hemorrhage and ulceration. *In vitro* and *in vivo* experiments had showed immunosuppressive properties at high dosages of patulin (Wouter & Speijers, 1996).

The International Agency for Research on Cancer (IARC) concluded that no evaluation was made respecting the carcinogenicity of patulin to humans and that there was inadequate evidence in experimental animals (IARC, 1986).

Even though no epidemic outbreak in humans and animals has been attributed to patulin contamination, increasing concern with public health forced the regulating authorities to establish maximum limits. As a consequence, international recommendations and regulations were established for patulin maximum levels allowed in food products; patulin content warnings in food products have to be displayed, acting like quality markers. Within European countries the regulation (EC) No 1425/2003 was adopted and setting as maximum levels of 50 μg/L for fruit juices and derived products, 25 μg/L for solid apple products and 10 μg/L for juices and foods aimed for babies and young infants (Commission regulation (EC) No 1881/2006). Joint FAO/WHO Expert Committee on Food Additives (JECFA) also established the provisional maximum tolerable daily intake 0.4 μg/kg body mass/day (JECFA, 1995). Nowadays, the US Food and Drug Administration (FDA) limit patulin to 50 μg/L.

2.4 Analysis

Patulin analysis encompass several important steps: sampling, sample preparation, isolation and/or identification, quantitation and, sometimes, statistical evaluation. Each step is equally important to obtain good results to fulfill the analytical purpose.

Sampling includes deciding on sampling points and choosing a method to get appropriate amounts of samples, which can be solid or liquid with very different structural and chemical complexity.

2.4.1 Sample preparation techniques

Most of the time, sample preparation is necessary to isolate and/or concentrate patulin from sample matrices, having into account its chemical properties and the complexity of matrices. As mentioned before, patulin can be found in human food and beverages, animal feed, biological and environmental samples.

Matrix solid-phase dispersion (MSPD) was reported (Wu et al., 2008, 2009) as a suitable method to extract patulin from apples, A small portion of apple was blended homogeneously in a C_{18}-bonded silica solid support. After the washing step with hexane, patulin was extracted by elution with dichloromethane. After solvent evaporation, the extract was dissolved in acetic acid buffer solution and the patulin was analyzed by High Performance Liquid Chromatography (HPLC).

The Association of Official Analytical Chemists (AOAC) adopted a liquid-liquid extraction as sample preparation methodology for patulin analysis of apple juices and concentrates in its Official Method 995.10 (Sewram et al., 2000, as cited in Brause et al., 1996). The method includes an initial multi-extraction step with ethyl acetate and a posterior extraction with an aqueous sodium carbonate solution. The combined extracts were dried and evaporated, then being dissolved in acetic acid solution and chromatographed for patulin analysis. Several improved methodologies of the official method have been reported over the years (Gökmen & Acar, 1998; Iha & Sabino, 2006). One of them was described for cloudy apple juice and apple purees, and includes a pretreatment procedure with pectinase to improve the clarity of juices and purees before patulin analysis (MacDonald et al., 2000).

2.4.1.1 Solid Phase Extraction (SPE)

Solid phase extraction (SPE) emerged as an extremely attractive versatile technique for sample preparation of patulin containing matrices. The principles of the technique are based on chromatography: solutes are dissolved or suspended in a liquid and eluted through a solid phase; depending on their affinity, a separation occurs (Figure 3). SPE has been used to clean-up matrices and concentrate trace substances, such as patulin. Like any other technique it has also limitations: matrix effect and the undesired competition between analyte(s) and the other matrix components. As can be seen in Figure 3, SPE uses pre-packed cartridges containing up to 500 mg of stationary phase - silica or silica bonded to specific functional groups such as hydrocarbons of variable chain length, reversed phase SPE, or quaternary ammonium or amino groups, anion-exchange SPE, or sulfonic acid or carboxylic groups, cation-exchange SPE.

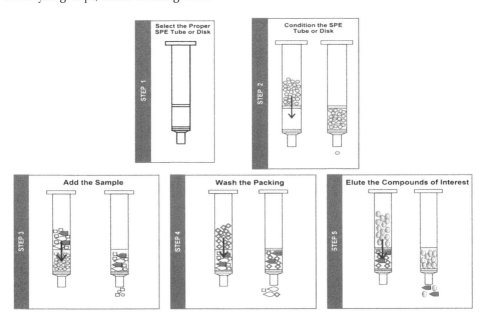

Fig. 3. SPE procedure steps (Supelco, 1998).

For patulin analysis in apple juices (Gökmen et al., 2005) two SPE systems using a tandem polyvinylpolypyrrolidone-octadecyl (PVPP-C18) cartridge and a hydrophilic lipophilic balanced (HLB) macroporous copolymer sorbent cartridge, were described. The technique required few mL of juice and the elution was done with diethyl ether. After solvent evaporation the residue was dissolved in a mixture of acetonitrile/water with a small portion of acetic acid and then chromatographed.

Another work reported the patulin analysis of infant's apple-based products involving a SPE cleanup step using a unconditioned silica gel cartridge (Arranz et al., 2005).

For the analysis of an apple juice syrup it was described a pretreatment procedure using C_{18}-SPE cartridges (Li et al., 2007). The syrup sample was diluted with acetic acid buffer solution and loaded onto the column. After the washing procedure using hexane, the cartridge was dried with a strong stream of air for 15 min, and eluted with the solvent mixture (hexane/ethyl acetate/acetone) in a gradient mode. After acidification, patulin was analyzed by HPLC.

2.4.1.2 Microextraction by packed sorbent or packaged syringe (MEPS)

The development of miniaturized analytical techniques has been done to fulfill many requirements and also enable rapid analysis at lower operation costs, with lower environmental pollution problems. Microextraction by packed sorbent or packaged syringe (MEPS) methodology seems to be a very promising solution in patulin analysis. MEPS technique uses a small amount of stationary phase, packed in the drum called BIN (Barrel Insert and Needle Assembly, Figure 4) of a gastight syringe (100μL – 250μL). Like SPE, MEPS aims the elimination of interferences and the selective isolation and concentration of the target compounds, but in a micro scale. MEPS procedure steps are similar to SPE laboratorial approaches and are illustrated in Figure 5.

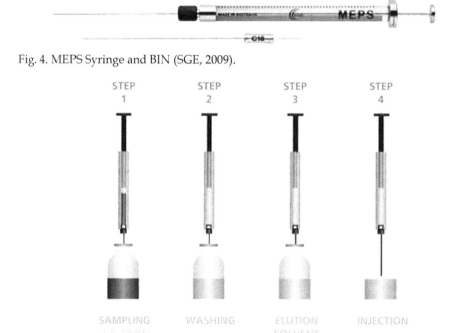

Fig. 4. MEPS Syringe and BIN (SGE, 2009).

Fig. 5. MEPS procedure steps (SGE, 2009).

Using MEPS as sample preparation technique, a new methodology for patulin analysis is described, for the first time, in this book chapter (Section 2.4.3.2). It aims the identification and quantification of this mycotoxin in real matrices.

2.4.2 Chromatographic methodologies

The most suitable analytical methods respecting accuracy, low detection limits and simple procedures for patulin analysis in food products, especially apple juice and its derivatives, involve chromatographic techniques such as thin-layer chromatography (TLC), gas chromatography (GC) and high-performance liquid chromatography (HPLC).

The pioneering methodology used in the identification and quantification of patulin, in apple juice, was thin-layer chromatography (TLC) with the advantages of being simple and low cost. One official method of the Association of Official Analytical Chemists (AOAC) for the analysis of mycotoxins (1974) uses TLC followed by silica gel column chromatography as sample preparation procedures. The analysis was carried out in silica gel plates, using, for detection, the reaction of patulin with 3-methyl-2-hydrazone benzothiazolinone and HCl (MBTH). The limit of detection (LOD) was described as 20 µg/L (Shephard & Leggott, 2000, as cited in Scott, 1974). Alternative detection and quantification methods were described using fluorodensiometry (Shephard & Leggott, 2000, as cited in Duraković et al., 1993), or absorbance–transmittance followed by densitometry at 275nm (Shephard & Leggott, 2000, as cited in Leming et al., 1993). Reversed phase TLC was also investigated, but despite the patulin elution with a wide variety of solvents, the technique was not applied to contaminated samples (Shephard & Leggott, 2000).

HPLC coupled with ultraviolet (UV) or photodiodes (DAD) detection is the most used chromatographic technique for patulin analysis; it allows an easy identification and quantification of patulin through its characteristic absorption spectrum. The AOAC also adopted HPLC-UV method (official method 995.10), for the detection and quantification of patulin in apple juices. As mentioned before, liquid-liquid extraction was used as sample preparation technique. The HPLC was done using a C_{18} reversed phase column, with particle size of 5 µm and pore size ranging from 12 to 25 nm, and isocratic elution with a flow of 1mL/min, and the eluent was composed by acetonitrile in acidified water. UV detection at 276 nm (Moake et al., 2005, as cited in AOAC official method 995.10) was used. The LOD achieved is low (5 µg/L).

Improved AOAC methods were described in the literature for the determination of patulin in apple juices (Gökmen & Acar, 2005) and in apple solid derivatives (Katerere et al., 2008). Over the years, HPLC methodologies associated with mass spectrometry (MS) were also developed. A work published in 2000 described patulin detection by collision-induced dissociation (CID) using atmospheric pressure chemical ionization (APCI); the LOD was good, with values near 4 µg/L (Sewram et al., 2000).

Gas chromatography (GC) has also been applied in the analysis of patulin. The literature reported GC-MS analysis by electron impact ionization, using a silylated patulin derivative (Moukas et al., 2008). Raw patulin (not derivatized) was also determined in apple juice by GC-MS using negative chemical ionization (Roach et al., 2000). Other GC methods were reported using on-column injection and selected ion monitoring (SIM) detection (Moake et al., 2005, as cited in Llovera et al., 1999).

A protocol including biphasic dialysis extraction, *in situ* acylation, as sample preparation and GC-MS (SIM) analysis was developed for detection and quantification of patulin (acetylated) in fruit juices (Sheu & Shyu, 1999). Another work presented the detection and quantification of C^{13} labeled patulin (Rychlik & Schieberle, 1999).

Capillary electrophoresis (CE) was also described as an alternative method for patulin analysis. In 2000, a capillary electrophoresis method was published as an analytical tool for rapid and highly sensitive analysis of patulin in cider; a fused silica capillary column was used, and the elution was done with an aqueous. The separation was achieved by migration of charged particles in the buffer. The cations migrated to the cathode and anions migrated to the anode under the influence of an electro-osmotic flow (EOF). In fact, compounds or mixtures of neutral and charged compounds can be analyzed by micellar electrokinetic capillary electrophoresis or micellar electrokinetic capillary chromatography (MECC). The method was described as having the advantage of requiring small amounts of sample and smaller amount of organic solvents when compared with HPLC (Tsao & Zhou, 2000).

2.5 Development of improved analytical methodologies

For patulin analysis, two sample preparation procedures using SPE and MEPS were developed and associated with an improved reversed-phase HPLC methodology (Gaspar & Lucena, 2009). The purpose was to simplify the sample, liberating the patulin from its original matrix, and allowing therefore a better performance of the overall analytical method. Table 1 shows the analytical parameters of the HPLC methodology.

Retention time (min)	Linearity			LOD (µg/L)	LOQ (µg/L)	Precision (RSD,%), n = 4
	Range (mg/L)	Calibration equation	R^2			
16.8	0.03 – 0.50	y = 136592x-2161.5	0.9996	2.0	6.0	3.5

Table 1. Analytical parameters of improved HPLC methodology for patulin analysis (Elvira & Lucena, 2009).

2.5.1 SPE-HPLC/DAD methodology

Aiming a small scale sample preparation procedure, a previously described SPE approach (Li et al., 2007) was improved and optimized. The purpose was the analysis of patulin in fresh fruits, namely apples, but also in apple juices commercialized in Portugal. The SPE sample preparation optimization was done by spiking fresh (healthy) apples extracts with patulin, in order to establish the best SPE analytical conditions, such as the choice of stationary phase and its conditioning, washing and extraction steps.

The SPE optimized sequential procedure is:

1. Using C_{18}-SPE cartridges, pre-washed with (3 mL) methanol, methanol:water (3 mL, 10% methanol) and acidified water (3 mL MilliQ water-perchloric acid ((100): 0.01,(v/v))) sequentially (illustrated in Figure 3, steps 1 and 2);
2. The column was not allowed to run dry;

3. The sample (0.5 mL) was introduced and eluted at a flow rate of 2–3 mL/min (Figure 3, step 3);
4. The following washing step was done with (0.5 mL) acidified water (Figure 3, step 4);
5. Sample elution was done with (3 × 1 mL) methanol (Figure 3, step 5);
6. The combined eluates were evaporated to dryness under vacuum;
7. After dissolution in (0.5 mL) acidified water the sample was analyzed using the previously mentioned improved HPLC methodology (Gaspar & Lucena, 2009);

This improved sample preparation changed the previously described (Li et al., 2007) washing solvent - acidified water instead of hexane - and also the eluent composition, methanol, a greener solvent, instead of the mixture hexane/ethyl acetate/acetone.

This optimized SPE-HPLC/DAD methodology showed an average recovery of 82% with a RSD value of 6% in the linear dynamic range 200 to 600 ppb (Table 2). The precision of the method showed a repeatability of 1.2% and a reproducibility value of 2.2%. According to the literature (Miller & Miller, 1988; IPQ, 2000) being these values below 10%, they indicate a good method performance. The overall SPE-HPLC methodology represents an economical, faster and routine usable methodology.

Range (µg/L)	Recovery (RSD,%), n = 3	Repeatability (RSD,%), n = 3	Reproducibility (RSD,%), n = 3
200 - 600	82 (6)	1.2	2.2

Table 2. Analytical parameters of improved SPE-HPLC methodology for patulin analysis.

2.5.2 MEPS-HPLC/DAD methodology

Using the recent MEPS analytical tool (Abdel-Rehim, 2004), a new, simple, sample preparation method was developed for patulin analysis. MEPS methodology can be rationalized as a miniaturization of SPE analytical system; it employs smaller quantities of sample and eluent (few microliters), being also adequate to remove interferences, simplifying the analysis.

For patulin analysis, this new sample preparation methodology was performed using the following sequential steps:

1. MEPS was carried out by means of a SGE Analytical Science (SGE Analytical Science, Germany) apparatus, consisting of a 250 µL HPLC syringe with a removable needle; the syringe was fitted with a BIN (Barrel Insert and Needle) containing the C_{18} sorbent and was used to draw and discharge samples and solutions through the BIN (Figure 4);
2. The sorbent was activated/conditioned three times with (3 × 100 µL) methanol and (5 × 100 µL) MilliQ water-perchloric acid ((100): 0.01 (v/v)) (Figure 5);
3. Sampling was done using a volume of 2x25 µL of sample solution, being introduced through the stationary phase for three times, in order to remove the interferences and retain the patulin (illustrated in Figure 5, step 1);
4. The analyte was eluted using methanol (2 × (3 × 25 µL)) and after analyzed by HPLC using the previously described conditions (Gaspar & Lucena, 2009) (illustrated in Figure 5, steps 3 and 4);

This method development evidenced the relevance of several factors in this sample preparation methodology, MEPS: sampling speed was around 10 µL/s, sample introduction was done in a fractionated mode (2 × 25 µL) and the washing step was not used; these procedures revealed a better recovery. The extracting solvent was of crucial importance - methanol was much better than acetonitrile for the patulin analysis.

The method performance was achieved using five replicates, spiking the target samples (apples) with different quantities of patulin standard ranging from 200 to 600 ppb (Table 3). The average recovery was 69% with a RSD of 4%. The precision of the method showed a repeatability of 3.2% and a reproducibility value of 4.0%. Also here these values are below 10%, indicating a good precision for this new sample preparation methodology (Miller & Miller, 1988; IPQ, 2000). MEPS can be an excellent alternative to the SPE technique, being faster, less solvent consuming and less expensive than SPE.

Range (µg/L)	Recovery (RSD,%), n = 5	Repeatability (RSD,%), n = 5	Reproducibility (RSD,%), n = 3
200 - 600	69 (4)	3.2	4.0

Table 3. Analytical parameters of MEPS-HPLC methodology for patulin analysis.

2.5.3 Analysis of food matrices

Two food matrices: an infected apple and a commercial apple juice were analyzed using both sample preparation methodologies: SPE-HPLC/DAD and MEPS-HPLC/DAD. These analyses are shown in Figures 6 and 7.

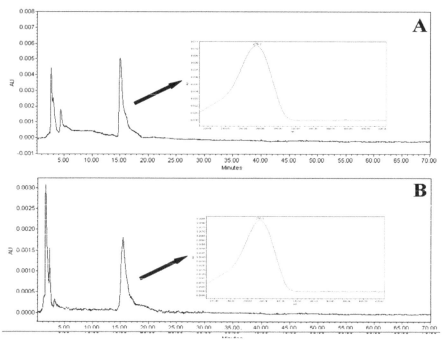

Fig. 6. SPE-HPLC/DAD (A) and MEPS-HPLC/DAD (B) patulin analysis from a naturally infected apple; the UV spectrum is shown (conditions described in Section 2.4.3.1 and 2.4.3.2).

As it was mentioned before, patulin is formed in bruised apples as a result of contamination with fungi. The analysis of an infected (mouldy) apple revealed that it contains a very high amount of patulin (894 ppm in SPE-HPLC/DAD and 919 ppm in MEPS-HPLC/DAD), much higher than its LD_{50} (5 mg/Kg = 5 ppm). This result indicates how dangerous is the direct consumption of damaged fruits and their use in the production of fruit juices (Figure 6).

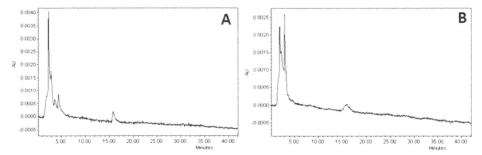

Fig. 7. SPE-HPLC/DAD (A) and MEPS-HPLC/DAD (B) patulin analysis from a spiked commercial apple juice; spike 7.7 ηg /50 μL (conditions described in Section 2.4.3.1 and 2.4.3.2).

Apple juice (cloudy) was also analysed by both methods showing a level of patulin lower than 6 ppb, the limit of quantification (LOQ) of both methods for this compound. Spiked matrices (Figure 7) were also analyzed, by both methods, to test the methodologies. The results revealed that the analyzed juice was produced with good sanitation criteria, satisfying the legislation limits (Commission Regulation (EC) No 1881/2006). These results show the necessity of constant surveillance of the occurrence of this toxin in fruit juices and evidenced that national public institutions should be capable of evaluating and determining food content in toxic substances in real time, due to the risk associated with consumption.

3. Conclusions

Patulin analysis is an important subject with social relevance. This chapter describes the most suitable analytical methods respecting accuracy, low detection limits and simple procedures for application in quality control, developed for the determination of patulin in food products, especially apple juice and its derivatives. Techniques such as thin-layer chromatography (TLC), gas chromatography (GC) and high-performance liquid chromatography (HPLC) were described together with sample preparation methodologies like liquid–liquid extraction (LLE) and solid-phase extraction (SPE) to determine the patulin. This chapter also describes, for the first time, an improved, simple, no time consuming, trace analysis micro extraction in packed syringe (MEPS) methodology for the determination of patulin in food products, and compares and discusses the use of MEPS and SPE in patulin extraction.

Having into account the importance of detecting this mycotoxin in food chain as marker of quality, this work will contribute to a better characterization and quantification of its presence in human diet and will make possible to determine the toxicological relevance of human exposure to patulin, its biological role and long-term implications of its consumption for human health.

4. Acknowledgements

Portuguese Foundation for Science and Technology is acknowledged for funding PhD grants: FCT SFRH/33809/2009 (Inês Nunes) and FCT SFRH/SFRH/BD/40564/2007 (João Lopes).

5. References

Abdel-Rehim, M. (2004) New trend in sample preparation: on-line microextraction in packed syringe for liquid and gas chromatography applications - I. Determination of local anaesthetics in human plasma samples using gas chromatography-mass spectrometry. *Journal of Chromatography B*, Vol.801, No.2, pp.317-321, 1570-0232

Abramson, D.; Mills, J.T.; Marquardt, R.R.; Frohlich, A.A. (1997) Mycotoxins in fungal contaminated samples of animal feed from western Canada, 1982-1994. *Canadian Journal of Veterinary Research*, Vol.61, No.1, pp.49-52, 0830-9000.

Arranz, I.; Derbyshire, M.; Kroeger, K.; Mischke, C.; Stroka, J.; Anklam, E. (2005) Liquid chromatographic method for quantitation of patulin at 10 ng/mL in apple-based products intended for infants: Interlaboratory study. *Journal of AOAC International*, Vol.88, No.2, pp.518-525, 1060-3271

Barreira, M.J.; Alvito, P.C.; Almeida, C.M.M. (2010) Occurrence of patulin in apple-based-foods in Portugal. *Food Chemistry*, Vol.121, No.3, pp.653-658, 0308-8146

Bennett, J.W. (1987). Mycotoxins, mycotoxicoses, mycotoxicology and Mycopathologia. *Mycopathologia*, Vol.100, No.1, pp.3-5, 0301-486X

Bennett, J.W.; Klich, M. (2003) Mycotoxins. *Clinical Microbiology Reviews*, Vol.16, No.3, pp.497-516, 0893-8512

Ciegler, A.; Detroy, R.W.; Lillehoj, E.B. (1971) Patulin, penicillic acid, and other carcinogenic lactones. in: *Microbial toxins*, Vol. 6, Ciegler, A; Kadis, S.; Ajl, S.J., pp.409-414, New York and London: Academic Press

Ciegler, A.; Beckwith, A.C.; Jackson, L.K. (1976) Teratogenicity of Patulin and Patulin Adducts Formed with Cysteine. *Applied and Environmental Microbiology*, Vol.31, No.5, pp.664-667, 0099-2240

Collin, S.; Bodart, E.; Badot, C.; Bouseta, A.; Nizet, S. (2008) Identification of the main degradation products of patulin generated through heat detoxication treatments. *Journal of the Institute of Brewing*, Vol.114, No.2, pp.167-171, 0046-9750

European Union. Commission Regulation (EC) No. 1881/2006 of 19 December 2006 setting maximum levels for certain contaminants in foodstuffs. *Official Journal of the European Union* L 364.

Gaspar, E.M.S.M.; Lucena, A.F.F. (2009) Improved HPLC methodology for food control - furfurals and patulin as markers of quality. *Food Chemistry*, Vol.114, No.4, pp.1576-1582, 0308-8146

Gökmen, V.; Acar, J. (1998) Incidence of patulin in apple juice concentrates produced in Turkey. *Journal of chromatography A*, Vol.815, No.1, pp.99-102, 0021-9673

Gökmen, V.; Acar, J.; Sarioglu, K. (2005) Liquid chromatographic method for the determination of patulin in apple juice using solid-phase extraction. *Analytica Chimica Acta*, Vol.543, No.1-2, pp.64-69, 0003-2670

IARC (1986) International Agency for Research on Cancer. Monographs on the evaluation of carcinogenic risk of chemicals to man, Vol. 40,pp.83, In: *INCHEM*, 24.06.2011, Available from: http://www.inchem.org/documents/iarc/vol40/patulin.html

Iha, M.H.; Sabino, M. (2006) Determination of patulin in apple juice by liquid chromatography. *Journal of AOAC International*, Vol.89, No.1, pp.139-143, 1060-3271

IPQ (2000) *Guia RELACRE 13 - Validação de métodos internos de ensaio em análise química*, Lisboa, Portugal

JECFA (1995) *Evaluation of certain food additives and contaminants: forty-fourth report of the Joint FAO/WHO Expert Committee on Food Additives*, WHO Technical Report Series No.859, 9241208597, Geneva

Katerere, D.R.; Stockenstrom, S.; Shephard, G.S. (2008) HPLC-DAD method for the determination of patulin in dried apple rings. *Food Control*, Vol.19, No.4, pp.389-392, 0956-7135

Katzman, P.A.; Hays, E.E.; Cain, C.K.; Van Wyk, J.J.; Reithel, F.J.; Thayer, S.A.; Doisy, E.A.; Gaby, W.L.; Carroll, C.J.; Muir, R.D.; Jones, L.R.; Wade, N.J. (1944) Clavacin, an antibiotic substance from Aspergillus Clavatus. *Journal of Biological Chemistry*, Vol.154, No.2, pp.475-486, 0021-9258

Krska, R.; Schubert-Ullrich, P.; Molinelli, A.; Sulyok, M.; Macdonald, S.; Crews, C. (2008) Mycotoxin analysis: An update. *Food Additives and Contaminants*, Vol.25, No.2, pp. 152-163, 0265-203X

Leggott, N.L.; Shephard, G.S. (2001) Patulin in South African commercial apple products. *Food Control*, Vol. 12, No.2, pp.73 – 76, 0956-7135

Li, J.K.; Wu, R.N.; Hu, Q.H.; Wang, J.H. (2007) Solid-phase extraction and HPLC determination of patulin in apple juice concentrate. *Food Control*, Vol.18, No.5, pp.530-534, 0956-7135

MacDonald, S.; Long, M.; Gilbert, J.; Felgueiras, I. (2000) Liquid chromatographic method for determination of patulin in clear and cloudy apple juices and apple puree: Collaborative study. *Journal of AOAC International*, Vol.83, No.6, pp.1387-1394, 1060-3271

Medical Research Council (2004) Clinical trial of patulin in the common cold. 1944. *International Journal of Epidemiology*, Vol.33, No.2, pp. 243-246, 0300-5771

Miller, J. C.; Miller, J. N. (1988) *Statistics for Analytical Chemistry* (Second Edition), Ellis Horwood: Chichester, 0138454213

Moake, M.M.; Padilla-Zakour, O.I.; Worobo, R.W. (2005) Comprehensive review of patulin control methods in foods. *Comprehensive Reviews in Food Science and Food Safety*, Vol.4, No.1, pp.8-21, 1541-4337

Moukas, A.; Markaki, P.; Panagiotopoulou, V. (2008) Determination of patulin in fruit juices using HPLC-DAD and GC-MSD techniques. *Food Chemistry*, Vol.109, No.4, pp.860-867, 0308-8146

Nielsen, K.F.; Smedsgaard, J. (2003) Fungal metabolite screening: Database of 474 mycotoxins and fungal metabolites for dereplication by standardised liquid chromatography-UV-mass spectrometry methodology. *Journal of Chromatography A*, Vol.1002, No.1-2, pp.111-136, 0021-9673

Peraica, M.; Radic, B.; Lucic, A.; Pavlovic, M. (1999) Toxic effects of mycotoxins in humans. *Bulletin of the World Health Organization*, Vol.77, No.9, pp.754-766, 0042-9686

Roach, J.A.G.; White, K.D.; Trucksess, M.W.; Thomas, F.S. (2000) Capillary gas chromatography/mass spectrometry with chemical ionization and negative ion detection for confirmation of identity of patulin in apple juice. *Journal of AOAC International*, Vol.83, No.1, pp.104-112, 1060-3271

Robbins, C.A.; Swenson, L.J.; Neally, M.L.; Kelman, B.J.; Gots, R.E. (2000) Health Effects of Mycotoxins in Indoor Air: A Critical Review. *Applied Occupational and Environmental Hygiene*, Vol.15, No.10, pp.773-784, 1047-322X

Rychlik, M.; Schieberle, P. (1999) Quantification of the mycotoxin patulin by a stable isotope dilution assay. *Journal of Agricultural and Food Chemistry*, Vol.47, No.9, pp. 3749-3755, 0021-8561

Sands, D.C.; Mcintyre, J.L.; Walton, G.S. (1976) Use of Activated-Charcoal for Removal of Patulin from Cider. Applied and Environmental Microbiology, Vol.32, No.3, pp.388-391, 0099-2240

Sant'Ana, A.D.; Rosenthal, A.; de Massaguer, P.R. (2008) The fate of patulin in apple juice processing: A review. *Food Research International*, Vol.41, No.5, pp.441-453, 0963-9969

Scott, P.M.; Toft, P.; Miles, W.F.; Dube, J.G. (1972) Occurrence of Patulin in Apple Juice. *Journal of Agricultural and Food Chemistry*, Vol.20, No.2, pp.450-451, 0021-8561

SGE (2009) MEPS™, In: *SGE Analytical Science*, 28.06.2011, Available from:
http://www.sge.com/products/meps
http://www.sge.com/uploads/3a/2f/3a2f95cbbb22cd8e8e3f2217220d48aa/LR_B R-0238-M.pdf

Sewram, V.; Nair, J.J.; Nieuwoudt, T.W.; Leggott, N.L.; Shephard, G.S. (2000) Determination of patulin in apple juice by high-performance liquid chromatography-atmospheric pressure chemical ionization mass spectrometry. *Journal of Chromatography A*, Vol.897, No.1-2, pp.365-374, 0021-9673

Shephard, G.S.; Leggott, N.L. (2000) Chromatographic determination of the mycotoxin patulin in fruit and fruit juices. *Journal of Chromatography A*, Vol.882, No.1-2, pp.17-22, 0021-9673

Shephard, G.S. (2008) Determination of mycotoxins in human foods. *Chemical Society Reviews*, Vol.37, No.11, pp.2468-2477, 0306-0012

Sheu, F.; Shyu, Y.T. (1999) Analysis of patulin in apple juice by diphasic dialysis extraction with in situ acylation and mass spectrometric determination. *Journal of Agricultural and Food Chemistry*, Vol.47, No.7, pp.2711-2714, 0021-8561

Sommer, N.F.; Buchanan, J.R.; Fortlage, R.J. (1974) Production of Patulin by Penicillium-Expansum. *Applied Microbiology*, Vol.28, No.4, pp.589-593, 0003-6919

Songsermsakul, P.; Razzazi-Fazeli, E. (2008) A review of recent trends in applications of liquid chromatography-mass spectrometry for determination of mycotoxins. *Journal of Liquid Chromatography & Related Technologies*, Vol.31, No.11-12, pp.1641-1686, 1082-6076

Supelco (1998) Guide to Solid Phase Extraction, Bulletin 910, In: *Sigma Aldrich*, 27.06.2011, Available from:
http://www.sigmaaldrich.com/Graphics/Supelco/objects/4600/4538.pdf

Tsao, R.; Zhou, T. (2000) Micellar electrokinetic capillary electrophoresis for rapid analysis of patulin in apple cider. *Journal of Agricultural and Food Chemistry*, Vol.48, No.11, pp. 5231-5235, 0021-8561

Wouters, M.F.A. and G.J.A. Speijers,(1996) Patulin. Food additives series 35. Toxicological evaluation of certain food additives and contaminants. In: *World Health Organisation*, Geneva, Switzerland, 24.06.2011, Available from: http://www.inchem.org/documents/jecfa/jecmono/v35je16.htm

Wu, R.N.; Dang, Y.L.; Niu, L.; Hu, H. (2008) Application of matrix solid-phase dispersion-HPLC method to determine patulin in apple and apple juice concentrate. *Journal of Food Composition and Analysis*, Vol.21, No.7, pp.582-586, 0889-1575

Wu, R.N.; Han, F.L.; Shang, J.; Hu, H.; Han, L. (2009) Analysis of patulin in apple products by liquid-liquid extraction, solid phase extraction and matrix solid-phase dispersion methods: a comparative study. *European Food Research and Technology*, Vol.228, No.6, pp.1009-1014, 1438-2377

4

Utilization of Marine Crustaceans as Study Models: A New Approach in Marine Ecotoxicology for European (REACH) Regulation

Pane Luigi, Agrone Chiara, Giacco Elisabetta,
Somà Alessandra and Mariottini Gian Luigi
DIP.TE.RIS, University of Genova, Genova,
Italy

1. Introduction

During last decades the productive activities, the increasing energy demand and the massive resource exploitation have caused extensive pollution phenomena that are to date spread on a worldwide scale. Therefore, the monitoring and assessment of environmental pollution is a subject of high concern owing to the implications that pollutants can exert on the environment, organisms and ecosystems, as well as on the quality of life of humans and on public health.

Pollution problems affect greatly the aquatic environments that are mainly sensitive to several typologies of contamination, such as chemical pollution, oil dumping, microbiological contamination from sewers, etc. These inputs can exert devastating effects on ecosystems with long-term consequences (Mille et al., 1998).

To date a lot of chemicals are utilized in productive processes and many new substances are synthesized every year; the utilization and introduction of these newly synthesized chemicals into the environment and in production cycles must be approved after an accurate evaluation of their eventual toxic properties against selected organisms with the main purpose to protect the safety of plants and animals and the human health. To do this several experiments useful to test the effects consequent to contact, inhalation and ingestion and to estimate the risks connected to the acute/chronic exposition in the natural and work environments have been proposed with the aim to define some fundamental parameters, such as the acceptable dose, the risk dose, the lethal dose, etc.

These evaluations need to be carried out using test-species which are representative of the environmental compartment under consideration; in this connection, the availability of test-species able to furnish reliable and cheap results and to evaluate the activity of pollutants at the individual and ecosystem level is essential. Nevertheless, it is known that the tests on animals have ethical implications and often show problems connected to the reliability and to the application of results to the natural conditions. As a matter of fact, the test-organisms have their own physical, biological and biochemical characteristics and thus they can metabolize some substances, and suffer their effects, in a different way from each other and, in particular, differently from humans.

To date the availability of test-species, easy to collect and to rear, and sensitive to different xenobiotics, is an important aspect in ecotoxicology in order to characterize the risk of chemicals. In general, in toxicity tests some organisms belonging to a target-species are exposed, in controlled conditions, to the activity of the samples to be investigated (water, sediments, soil, sewage, sludge, chemicals, known toxicants, etc) in order to evaluate the eventual toxic effects. At the end of tests lethality or sub-lethality can be observed according to the considered end-point (mortality, growth, motility, physiological and reproductive alterations, etc.) and as a consequence of the utilized species and of the extent of measurable effect; furthermore, acute or chronic toxicity can be distinguished according to the duration of the test compared with the life cycle of the organism.

It is well known that different species have different ecological and biological characteristics; for this reason, to achieve an adequate description of the environmental injury using a single species is not possible in the laboratory. For this reason, the preparation of batteries of tests including some different species is a suitable procedure; selected species should be used in the tests on the basis of criteria useful to satisfy most of the requirements to correctly perform the ecotoxicological assessment.

Overall, the criteria useful to choose different test-species should comprise: the different phylogenetical position and trophic level, the different ecological relevance, the sensitivity to specific contaminants, the relative shortness of the life cycle, the easy availability, the known adaptation to laboratory conditions, the possibility to respond to the different ways of exposition to contaminants. Furthermore, the main requirements of a toxicological test can be summarized as: standardization, possibility to give replicates, easy realization, possibility to discriminate between different results, cost reduction, rapidity of execution (Onorati & Volpi Ghirardini, 2001).

In the aquatic environment an ideal battery of organisms should comprise the representative links of the food web: a primary producer, such as a microalga, a primary consumer (invertebrate), such as a crustacean, and a secondary consumer (vertebrate), such as a fish (Shaw & Chadwick, 1995), taking into account the specific application, the typology of the considered environment, the presumptive levels of pollutants, the physico-chemical characteristics of the involved substances, the purpose of the ecotoxicological study, as well as the available resources.

In this connection, the new European regulation REACH (Registration, Evaluation, Authorization of Chemicals) No. 1907/2006 introduces an integrated system for the management of all produced/imported chemicals for an amount ≥1 ton/year and states that all substances destined to be used in the EU and to be introduced into the production processes must be subject to accurate evaluation including toxicity tests on selected organisms.

All tests indicated by REACH must be carried out in conformity with well defined analysis methods determined by the EU or, failing that, according to the OECD guidelines or to other determined methods. Furthermore, all tests must be performed in conformity with the principles of Good Laboratory Practice (GLP) according to the pertinent Community directive.

2. A global view on reach regulation

The REACH regulation supplies information concerning what test must be performed to evaluate chemicals in different situations.

Acute toxicity tests concern the evaluation of adverse effects which can be observed after a short-term exposition (hours or days according to the utilized species); these tests should be carried out applying the OECD guidelines.

The repeated exposition can be distinguished in I) the sub-acute (or sub-chronic) one that concerns the studies with a daily exposition to chemicals of longer duration than acute ones, but not exceeding a defined part of the life span of the organism; for example, for fish species it must not exceed a period equivalent to one-third of the time taken to reach sexual maturity (Solbé, 1998) and II) the chronic one that concerns an exposition extending for all or for most of organism life span. The adverse effects of expositions concern the alterations of morphology, physiology, growth, development, reproduction and survival.

The reproductive toxicity concerns the effects on reproduction and fertility in adults and the development toxicity studies the effects on offspring. These tests are characterized by multiple endpoints which consider the reproductive disability or harmful non-hereditary effects on offspring. The REACH regulation provides for a screening test, a prenatal toxicity test (on one or two species) and a reproduction toxicity test for two generations. These tests should be carried out according to OECD methods.

Mutagenic, clastogenic and carcinogenic effects with permanent and transmissible changes of genetic material, structural chromosome aberration, change of chromosome number and genotoxic effects concern processes able to change the structure of DNA and the genetic information.

Degradation/biodegradation and bioconcentration/bioaccumulation are also considered in REACH regulation, with the advice to use OECD or other alternative methods. These studies are carried out on aquatic organisms as well as, in some situations, also on soil organisms such as earthworms and seeds.

2.1 Aquatic toxicity

The aquatic toxicity of chemicals is one of main aspects of REACH regulation and an important parameter for the evaluation of substances. As a matter of fact, water is the principal constituent of all living beings and in most of them it constitutes more than 70% of wet-weight. A lot of energy transfers, substance diffusion and enzyme reactions take place in waters; for this reason it has a pre-eminent biological concern. Therefore, the evaluation of the ecotoxicity on aquatic organisms is a fundamental step in the whole evaluation process of a chemical.

In ecotoxicity testing the organisms are exposed to different concentrations of chemicals/contaminants that can be assumed through respiration or teguments; then the balance repartition mechanisms between water and absorption compartments take place with the result of a progressive increase of the toxicant into the body (bioconcentration). After absorption the toxicant is subject to the distribution and to metabolic processes as well as to excretion; for these reasons it is difficult to estimate the internal concentration of toxicants and conventionally the toxicity is quantified in terms of concentration of the substance in the medium (Gaggi, 1998; Paoletti et al., 1998). In particular in aquatic ecotoxicology, and mainly when the invertebrates are considered, it is very difficult to estimate the amount of toxicant assumed into the body; so, this parameter is unknown, but is known the concentration of the toxicant in the water. Anyhow, it should also be considered that to vertebrates (fish or mammals) the toxicant can be administered directly into the body (blood and/or muscle) and therefore its amount is certainly known. So, these two cases are remarkably different and in the first case we can express the results as LC_{50} (Lethal Concentration) while in the second one as LD_{50} (Lethal Dose).

The tests can be subdivided in acute and chronic. The acute toxicity concerns experiments carried out for hours or days and is generally expressed as LC_{50}, that corresponds to the concentration able to reduce the survival of exposed organisms up to 50%, or EC_{50}, that corresponds to the highlighting of an adverse measurable effect such as immobilization. The chronic toxicity regards a long-term exposition (weeks, months) and theoretically can be extended during the whole life cycle of the organisms; the current endpoints are the NOEC (No Observed Effect Concentration) and the LOEC (Lowest Observed Effect Concentration) that generally consider the survival, growth and reproduction. The regulation recommends to use standardized methods but also well described non-standardized protocols or modified methods can be acceptable.

2.2 Test-organisms in aquatic toxicity

In aquatic toxicity tests procariotic organisms, algae, plants and animals having particular characteristics are used as test-species. In general, a test-species must show a known sensitivity to a stress agent, so in the presence of this agent it will suffer alterations of life functions, growth inhibition, reproductive and metabolic disorders or, on the contrary, it can find favourable conditions and develop to the prejudice of other species. It follows that to elect a species to the role of test-species is not easy because each species has its own sensitivity and therefore furnishes a different response (Calamari et al., 1980).

A fundamental factor is the "basic" knowledge of the test-species, that implies the knowledge of life cycle, natural mortality rate of the population and mortality rate of the first stages in order to avoid interferences with the mortality due to the toxic stress. As concerns the response it is necessary to consider that generally species that can survive and reproduce in various environmental conditions are more tolerant to toxicants than species adapted to live in defined conditions.

The research concerning the employment of animal organisms in ecotoxicology have had a remarkable impulse during the last two decades and several species have been used in ecotoxicological tests; so, the list of species that have been proposed to have a role in ecotoxicology is very long and is still in progress.

To date in ecotoxicology the principle that the potential toxicity of a substance can be evaluated only with batteries of ecotoxicity tests is accepted. Each battery must have at least three test-species with well defined life-stages; overall, the test should be carried out considering the different levels of the food web; therefore, it is essential to use a primary producer, such as an unicellular alga, a primary consumer, such as a filter feeder invertebrate, and a secondary consumer, such as larval fish. Also a saprotroph/saprophyte and a detritus-feeder should be comprised among the considered species (Baudo et al., 2011). Useful results could be also obtained through *in vitro* systems, such as cell cultures of fish cells (Pane & Mariottini, 2009). Finally, the test battery should have a good sensitivity and a discriminating potentiality in order to respond as much as possible to pollutants (Baudo et al., 2011).

Among aquatic organisms crustaceans have a key-role in the environment for their intermediate position in the food web and also for their wide distribution and high density; for this reason in ecotoxicological testing several crustacean species have been proposed (APHA, AWWA, WEF, 1995) and are having a wide employment both in freshwater and in marine ecotoxicology.

3. Utilization of crustaceans in ecotoxicology

Small crustaceans are an important link within the food web, playing an important role as primary consumers and sometimes also as secondary consumers, so they are eligible to be used in ecotoxicological evaluations; as a matter of fact, they connect the energetic fluxes between the primary producers (mainly algae) and the consumers of higher levels (such as fishes) and, therefore, they are placed at a key-level into the food web. To date only the freshwater cladoceran *Daphnia magna* is approved as suitable crustacean for aquatic tests in freshwater ecotoxicology.

3.1 Freshwater crustaceans

Daphnia magna is the most important test-species in freshwater ecotoxicology (Persoone & Janssen, 1998). The parthenogenetical reproduction in *Daphnia* allows to have identical specimens useful for testing. During the parthenogenesis females produce unfertilised eggs from which hatch only females. During adverse environmental conditions (extreme temperatures, increase of population density, accumulation of excretion products, low food availability) also males are produced; these males fertilize particular eggs (resting eggs) that are then carried by females into a particular structure known as 'ephippium'. From these eggs hatch females that will reproduce again parthenogenetically.

Daphnia magna is utilized essentially because it is widely distributed in freshwaters and constitutes an important link in the food web being placed at an intermediate position between primary producers and fish consumers; furthermore, in some small ecosystems it is the final consumer (Müller, 1980). The breeding of *Daphnia magna* in the laboratory is easy and, thanks to its biological characteristics, it is possible to obtain easily a lot of specimens homogeneous for age and growth rate. Furthermore, thanks to the parthenogenesis it is possible to have identical individuals; this is a very important factor to minimize the individual variations in the response to toxicants. In addition, *Daphnia magna* has a quite short life cycle, thus it is possible to carry out fast chronic toxicity tests also for more generations.

In toxicity test with *Daphnia magna* two main parameters, mortality and immobilization, are recorded and the results are expressed respectively as LC_{50} and EC_{50}. Nevertheless, the parameter "immobilization" has been subject of criticism because a scarce mobility was observed in "sluggish" specimens which were motionless after stimulation, but subsequently can return to swim actively (Müller, 1980).

The tests with *Daphnia magna* must be carried out according to well-defined standards. According to IRSA-CNR (1994) the organisms must have homogeneous age (<24 hours), in general the tests should be conducted for 24-48 hours in static flux conditions, at 20°C and pH 7.5-8.5, with light-dark period 16 hrs - 8 hrs; the utilized standard water must have total hardness 140-160 mg $CaCO_3$/l, alcalinity 110-120 mg $CaCO_3$/l.

Recent methods were published by OECD: the method OECD 202 (2004) concerns the use of young daphnids, aged less than 24 hrs, and the exposition to different concentrations of toxicants for 48 hrs against control test. The immobilisation must be evaluated after 24 and 48 hrs and the results must be expressed as EC_{50}. Other daphnid species, such as *Daphnia pulex*, *Ceriodaphnia affinis* and *Ceriodaphnia dubia*, can be utilized in this test. The method OECD 211 (2008) concerns the evaluation of reproduction and utilizes specimens aged less than 24 hrs. The exposition is prolonged for 21 days and the living offspring produced is evaluated; survival, LOEC and NOEC are the common expression of results.

3.2 Marine crustaceans

Marine crustaceans useful for ecotoxicological testing are both benthic and planktonic and can be chosen mainly from adult and larval copepods, larval brine shrimps, larval barnacles and amphipods.

On the whole, *Artemia*, the brine shrimp typical of hypersaline waters, has been considered for long time the "standard" species (Carli et al., 1998) and has been currently used to evaluate the acute toxicity of several inorganic and organic contaminants (Baudo et al., 2011). *Artemia* specimens are in general easily available and the breeding does not show particular difficulties; these are certainly important factors to promote the utilization of this organism. As a matter of fact, it is normally easy to obtain many individuals starting from commercial cysts. In spite of this, to date the employment of *Artemia* is controversial particularly owing to its supposed inadequate sensitivity (Weideborg et al., 1997; Davoren et al., 2005). Otherwise, recent studies indicated that the evaluation of survival in *Artemia* in long-term toxicity tests is an useful and sensitive parameter (Brix et al., 2003, 2004; Manfra et al., 2009).

In marine ecotoxicology some copepods, such as the calanoid *Acartia tonsa* and the harpacticoids *Nitocra spinipes*, *Tisbe battagliai*, *Tigriopus fulvus* and other *Tigriopus* spp., and the amphipods *Corophium insidiosus*, *Corophium orientale* and *Corophium volutator* and other species indicated by ASTM (1999) seem to be eligible to play the role of test-species (Baudo et al., 2011) in order to support the brine shrimp *Artemia*, already extensively used, and to replace not easily available species, such as the mysid *Mysidopsis bahia*, an autochthonous species of Eastern coasts of North America, that was indicated in some regulations without considering the difficulties of its importing in the EU.

Amphipods are widely used in ecotoxicology, owing to their sensitivity to several contaminants such as metals (Zanders & Rojas, 1992; Liber et al., 2011; Mann et al., 2011; Strom et al., 2011), for the evaluation of sediments in marine and transition environments

(Chapman & Wang, 2001) and have been employed to draw up sediment-quality guidelines (Macdonald et al., 2011).

ASTM (1999) suggests for testing some amphipods species but unfortunately none of them occurs in the Mediterranean, making problematical their use for the laboratories of this region; on the whole, among the species considered in the guidelines the sole amphipod useful for the Mediterranean is *Corophium orientale* that is cited in the protocol ISO 16712 (2005). *Corphium orientale* has been indicated to be suitable in ecotoxicology mainly for its constant availability, for its high tolerance to the variations of salinity and for the reproducibility of given results that were verified comparing different populations sampled in Italian sites (Lera et al., 2008) but, in spite of this, the difficulties in sampling and breeding is a critical factor. As a matter of fact, to date the main problem for using of these amphipods concerns the impossibility to breed them; among the European amphipods suggested by OSPAR (1995) only *Corophium volutator* has been bred in the laboratory (Peters & Ahlf, 2005), but it does not occur in the Mediterranean.

Otherwise, harpacticoid copepods can be useful test-organisms for their wide distribution, their key-position within the food web, their satisfactory sensitivity to pollutants and because they are easier to rear than other crustaceans and also than pelagic copepods. Furthermore, the breeding of some harpacticoids allows to have many organisms that are always available owing to the constant and abundant production of offspring with very low costs and efforts. In some harpacticoids the production of offspring can be also stimulated. For these reasons harpacticoid copepods seem to be the chief candidate to hold the role of primary consumer in ecotoxicological testings.

To date the studies on the ecotoxicological response of *Acartia tonsa* and *Tigriopus fulvus*, two species eligible to the role of test-species in aquatic ecotoxicology, are in progress in Italy with the aim to contribute to the standardization of test methodologies; these studies are being carried out in the framework of an Italian inter-calibration programme including different laboratories using heavy metals as reference substances.

4. New approaches in marine ecotoxicology: promising copepod test-species

Copepods are emergent organisms in ecotoxicology; to date their employment is increasing even though for some species the availability is a critical factor; the main problem concerns the adequacy of the test-species in relation to their environment.

As stated above, the copepods used in marine ecotoxicology are essentially the calanoid *Acartia tonsa* and the harpacticoids *Nitocra spinipes*, *Tisbe battagliai* and *Tigriopus fulvus*; other copepods have been used sporadically.

In spite of this, the usefulness of *Tisbe battagliai* and *Nitocra spinipes* can be problematical in the EU (Baudo et al., 2011).

The calanoid *Acartia tonsa* Dana, 1846 is a small euryhaline and eurytherm copepod, it is widely spread and is typical of eutrophic coastal waters and harbours, as well as of estuaries and lagoons worldwide (Cervetto et al., 1995). It is known to be a cosmopolitan copepod and occurs mainly in waters with high trophism (Baudo et al., 2011). In the Mediterranean region *Acartia tonsa* was found first in late '80s of the last century (Farabegoli et al., 1989; Sei et al., 1996); it is supposed to be an allochtonous species for the Mediterranean where to date occurs mainly in the Adriatic Sea.

Acartia tonsa can be found in all seasons, with remarkable abundance from April to November (Baudo et al., 2011). During the last decade it has been widely employed in toxicity testing with several substances such as metals (Bielmyer et al., 2006), endocrine disruptors (Andersen et al., 2001; Kusk & Wollenberger, 2007), brominated compounds (Wollenberger et al., 2005), cosmetic and sunscreen components (Kusk et al., 2011), LAS (linear alkyl benzene sulfonate) (Christoffersen et al., 2003), insecticides (Barata et al., 2002; Medina et al., 2002) and other different chemicals (Sverdrup et al., 2002).

The specimens useful for the experiments can be collected with zooplankton nets provided with 50 – 200 µm mesh; to start breeding it is suggested to collect 200-300 adult *Acartia tonsa* (both males and females). Adult males and females *Acartia tonsa* can be recognized under a dissecting microscope following the indications of classical taxonomy (Rose, 1933) and removed using a wide-bore pipette (Buskey & Hartline, 2003; Invidia et al., 2004). Zooplankton samples must be maintained in appropriate recipients at 20°C ± 0.5°C with aeration; the sorting of specimens and the taxonomical recognition must be carried out as soon as possible and anyhow within few days from sampling. Subsequently, *Acartia tonsa* can be maintained in flow-through system with natural seawater at temperature 20 ± 2°C; it is necessary to provide constant aeration and a light/dark period 16/8 hrs, at 1800-2100 lux (Widdows, 1998). The organisms can be fed twice a week *ad libitum* with algae from batch cultures of different species such as *Isochrysis galbana* and *Tetraselmis suecica*.

Algal cultures used to feed copepods must be used at the exponential growth phase; suitable density to feed copepods can be 1.3×10^6 cells/ml for *Isochrysis galbana* and 0.35×10^6 cells/ml for *Tetraselmis suecica* supplying 7 ml/l *Isochrysis galbana* and 7 ml/l *Tetraselmis suecica*. The counting of algal cells can be performed by using a Thoma hemocytometer.

Toxicity tests must be performed using *Acartia tonsa* eggs obtained 15-16 hours before the test starting from the specimens maintained in the laboratory at the above described conditions.

The harpacticoid copepod *Tigriopus fulvus* assumed recently a pre-eminent role in ecotoxicology and demonstrated to be a promising target-species (Todaro et al., 2001; Faraponova et al., 2003; Pane et al., 2006a, 2006b). *Tigriopus fulvus* is the most representative organism in the splashpools of rocky Mediterranean littorals (Pane & Mariottini, 2010); it is adapted to live in pools located at different height above the tideline, characterized by wide salinity variations and also by mixing of marine and fresh waters, while it is absent in the pools reached by waves and in higher pools that receive almost exclusively the contribution of freshwater (Carli et al., 1995). Anyhow, as it is well known after observations in the laboratory, *Tigriopus fulvus* can survive normally both in natural and in artificial seawater (Carli et al., 1989a).

The specimens can be easily sampled in splashpools of rocky coasts; before testing they need to be acclimatized at least ten days at the laboratory conditions in filtered natural or artificial seawater at temperature 18.0±0.5 °C, 18 PSU (Practical Salinity Units) and neutral pH, with a 12/12 hrs light/dark period. The organisms must be fed once a week with algae from batch cultures (mainly *Tetraselmis suecica* or *Chlorella minutissima*) and bakers' yeast (*Saccharomyces cerevisiae*) counting the cells by a Thoma hemocytometer (Pane et al., 2008b).

The ecotoxicological tests can be carried out on adults (generally only females are used because in laboratory breeding they preponderate on males) and on the first larval stages (nauplii I-II) born in the laboratory culture; for tests on nauplii to have same-aged specimens is a very important factor in order to standardize the procedure. A simple method to obtain a suitable amount of same-aged nauplii provides for the isolation of carrying eggs females; subsequently the hatching of eggs must be stimulated by detaching egg sacs using fine needles after immobilization of females by soft filtration on membrane filters leaving a thin water film to avoid to damage them (Pane et al., 2006b). Detached egg sacs must be transferred into cell culture multiwell plates in seawater (18 PSU) and maintained at 18±0.5°C for 24 hours. Newborn nauplii (I-II stage) hatched by detached eggs, having the same age, can be utilized in toxicity tests.

The chronic tests on females, besides survival, consider also the production of egg sacs and of alive nauplii, so, they should be carried out preferably in multiwell plates with extractable polystyrene inserts provided with a membrane with pore mesh size 74 μm that allow to separate the females from offspring and to easily count the nauplii (Pane et al, 2008b).

Tigriopus fulvus has been extensively studied from the biological (Carli & Fiori, 1977; Carli et al., 1989a), biochemical (Carli et al., 1989b; Pane et al., 2003) and ecological point of view (Carli et al., 1993; Pane et al., 2000). Some studies have used this copepod to evaluate the toxicity of metals, surfactants, dispersants and other compounds of environmental concern (Giacco et al., 2006; Pane et al., 2007a, 2007b, 2008a, 2008b, 2009) in the framework of extensive experiments including the use of ecotoxicological test sets with several organisms (bacteria, algae, crustaceans, fish larvae).

Tigriopus fulvus has been recently included by the Italian Law among the species to be used to evaluate the suitability of natural or synthetic absorbent products and dispersants employed in seawaters for draining of oil hydrocarbon contamination (Gazzetta Ufficiale della Repubblica Italiana, 2011).

Other species of the genus *Tigriopus* have been considered for ecotoxicology: the first studies were made during the '70s and 80's of the last century when the effect of environmental contaminants, such as oil by-products, and pesticides was studied on *Tigriopus californicus* by Barnett and Kontogiannis (1975) and Antia et al., (1985) respectively, demonstrating the high adaptive capability of these copepods to the stress caused by xenobiotics.

Tigriopus brevicornis was utilized mainly to assess the toxicity of both essential and non-essential metals (Forget et al., 1998; Barka et al., 2001), considering also the detoxification processes (Barka, 2000, 2007) and the enzyme activity (Forget et al., 2003). Other studies concerned the effect of thermal shocks simulating the action of coastal nuclear power stations (Falchier et al., 1981) and the assessment of pesticide toxicity (Forget et al., 1998). Its role as water quality indicator has been also considered (Barka et al., 1997).

Tigriopus japonicus has been widely used in ecotoxicology and a lot of papers are available; recently the exposition to benzo(a)pyrene (Bang et al., 2009) and to alkylphenols (Hwang et al., 2010) was assessed on this copepod. Furthermore, the action of effluents in comparison with *Daphnia magna* (Kang et al., 2011), of metals (Ki et al., 2009; Kim et al., 2011; Kwok et al., 2008; Rhee et al., 2009) and the expression of glutathione S-transferase (Lee et al., 2007, 2008), the exposition to endocrine disruptors (Lee et al., 2006, Rhee et al., 2009) and to antifouling biocides (Kwok & Leung, 2005) have been also studied recently.

5. Conclusion

To date pollution rising from anthropogenic sources play an increasing environmental role. In addition, this phenomenon has an interest in all environments because pollution occurring in air, soil and freshwaters can be carried to seawaters and drained into coastal zones exerting toxicity on all organisms and persisting in time. Taking into account also the bioaccumulation processes, the monitoring of ecotoxicity is essential to determine the effects of pollutants at the global level. In this framework the availability of sensitive test-species is a very important aspect.

In this connection some crustaceans, for their wide distribution and for their key-position in the food web, have been proposed recently as test-species in ecotoxicology and the obtained results seem to be promising. In particular, the calanoid copepod *Acartia tonsa* and the harpacticoid copepod *Tigriopus fulvus* have shown to have several useful characteristics to play the role of test-species in ecotoxicology in the procedure of "risk assessment" concerning different chemicals.

In conclusion, in the framework of the REACH regulation further efforts are needing to adequate the research and the testing to the new regulations, taking also into account the need to prefer the use of invertebrates instead of vertebrates and, where possible, to replace the toxicity experiments with living organisms with alternative techniques, including analytical techniques useful for the screening of substances, predictive models and *in vitro* procedures.

6. References

Andersen H.R., Wollenberger L., Halling-Sørensen B. & Kusk K.O. (2001). Development of copepod nauplii to copepodites - a parameter for chronic toxicity including endocrine disruption. *Environmental Toxicology and Chemistry*, Vol. 20, No. 12 (December 2001), pp. 2821-2829, ISSN 0730-7268.

Antia N.J., Harrison P.J., Sullivan D.S. & Bisalputra T. (1985). Influence of the insecticide Diflubenzuron (Dimilin) on the growth of marine Diatoms and a Harpacticoid Copepod in culture. *Canadian Journal of Fisheries and Aquatic Sciences*, Vol. 42, No. 7 (July 1985), pp. 1272-1277, ISSN 0706-652X.

APHA, AWWA, WEF (American Public Health Association, American Water Works Association, Water Environment Federation) (1995). *Standard methods for the examination of water and wastewater*, Eaton A.D., Clesceri L.S., Greenberg A.E. (Eds.), American Public Health Association, Washington DC, USA.

ASTM (1999). Standard Guide for Conducting 10-Day Static Sediment Toxicity Tests With Marine and Estuarine Amphipods. ASTM E1367, pp. 1-27.

Bang H.W., Lee W. & Kwak I.-S. (2009). Detecting points as developmental delay based on the life-history development and urosome deformity of the harpacticoid copepod, *Tigriopus japonicus sensu lato*, following exposure to benzo(a)pyrene. *Chemosphere*, Vol. 76, No. 10 (2009), pp. 1435–1439, ISSN 0045-6535.

Barata C., Medina M., Telfer T. & Baird D.J. (2002). Determining demographic effects of
cypermethrin in the marine copepod *Acartia tonsa*: stage-specific short tests versus
life-table tests. *Archives of Environmental Contamination and Toxicology*, Vol. 43, No. 3
(October 2002), pp. 373-378, ISSN 0090-4341.

Barka, S. (2000). Processus de détoxication et localisation tissulaire des métaux traces
(cuivre, zinc, nickel, cadmium, argent et mercure) chez un crustacé marin *Tigriopus
brevicornis* (Müller). Etude du biomarqueur "protéines type métallothionéines", de
la bioaccumulation des métaux et des conséquences sur le transfert trophique.
Thése de Doctorat, Université de Paris 6, 19 septembre 2000, 204 p. + annexes.

Barka S. (2007). Insoluble detoxification of trace metals in a marine copepod *Tigriopus
brevicornis* (Müller) exposed to copper, zinc, nickel, cadmium, silver and mercury.
Ecotoxicology. Vol. 16, No. 7 (October 2007), pp. 491-502, ISSN 0963-9292.

Barka S., Forget J., Menasria M.R. & Pavillon J.F. (1997). Le copépode *Tigriopus brevicornis*
(Müller) peut-il étre considéré comme une sentinelle de la qualité de
l'environnement dans la zone supra-littorale? *Journal de Recherche Océanographique*,
Vol. 23, No. 4, pp. 131–138, ISSN 0397-5347.

Barka S., Pavillon J.-F. & Amiard J.-C. (2001). Influence of different essential and non-
essential metals on MTLP levels in the Copepod *Tigriopus brevicornis*. *Comparative
Biochemistry and Physiology Part C: Toxicology & Pharmacology*, Vol. 128, No. 4 (April
2001), Pp. 479-493, ISSN 1532-0456.

Barnett C.J. & Kontogiannis J.E. (1975). The effect of crude oil fractions on the survival of a
tidepool Copepod, *Tigriopus californicus*. *Environmental Pollution*, Vol. 8, No. 1, pp.
45-54, ISSN 0269-7491.

Baudo R., Faimali M., Onorati F. & Pellegrini D. (2011). *Batterie di saggi ecotossicologici per
sedimenti di acque salate e salmastre*. I manuali di Ecotossicologia, Manuali e linee
guida, ISPRA Istituto Superiore per la Protezione e la Ricerca Ambientale, 67/2011,
ISBN: 978-88-448-0498-5, Roma, Italy.

Bielmyer G. K., Grosell M. & Brix K. V. (2006). Toxicity of silver, zinc, copper and nickel to
the copepod *Acartia tonsa* exposed via a phytoplankton diet. *Environmental Science
and Technology*, Vol. 40, No. 6 (March 2006), pp. 2063-2068, ISSN 0013-936X.

Brix K.V., Cardwell R.D. & Adams W.J. (2003). Chronic toxicity of arsenic to the Great Salt
Lake brine shrimp, *Artemia franciscana*. *Ecotoxicology and Environmental Safety*, Vol.
54, No. 2 (February 2003), pp. 169-175, ISSN 0147-6513.

Brix K.V., Deforest D.K., Cardwell R.D. & Adams W.J. (2004). Derivation of a chronic site-
specific water quality standard for selenium in the Great Salt Lake, Utah, USA.
Environmental Toxicology and Chemistry, Vol. 23, No. 3 (March 2004), pp. 606-612,
ISSN 0730-7268.

Buskey E.J. & Hartline D.K. (2003). High-speed video analysis of the escape responses of the
Copepod *Acartia tonsa* to shadows. *Biological Bulletin*, Vol. 204, No. 1 (February
2003), pp. 28–37, ISSN 0006-3185.

Calamari D., Da Gasso R., Galassi S., Provini A. & Vighi M. (1980). Biodegradation and
toxicity of selected amines on aquatic organisms. *Chemosphere*, Vol. 9, No. 12, pp.
753-762, ISSN 0045-6535.

Carli A. & Fiori A. (1977). Morphological analysis of the two *Tigriopus* species found along
the European coasts (Copepoda Harpacticoida). Natura, Vol. 68, No. 1-2, pp. 101-
110.

Carli A., Mariottini G.L. & Pane L. (1989a). Reproduction of the rockpools harpacticoid
copepod *Tigriopus fulvus* (Fischer 1860), suitable for aquaculture. Deuxième

Congrès international d'Aquariologie (1988) Monaco, *Bulletin de l'Institut Océanographique de Monaco*, No. spécial 5, pp. 295-300, ISSN 0304-5722.

Carli A., Balestra V., Pane L. & Valente T. (1989b). Rapporto di composizione percentuale degli acidi grassi nel *Tigriopus fulvus* delle pozze di scogliera della costa ligure (Copepoda Harpacticoida). *Bollettino della Società Italiana di Biologia Sperimentale*, Vol. 65, No. 5, pp. 421-427, ISSN 0037-8771.

Carli A., Pane L., Casareto L., Bertone S. & Pruzzo C. (1993). Occurrence of *Vibrio alginolyticus* in Ligurian coast rock pools (Tyrrhenian Sea, Italy) and its association with the copepod *Tigriopus fulvus* (Fischer 1860). *Applied Environmental Microbiology*, Vol. 59, No. 6 (June 1993), pp. 1960-1962, ISSN 0099-2240.

Carli A., Feletti M. & Mariottini G.L. (1995). Problemi di adattamento in ambienti confinati: *Tigriopus fulvus* Fischer (Copepoda, Harpacticoida). *Biologi Italiani*, Vol. 25, No. 1 (January 1995), pp. 22-27, ISSN 0392-2510.

Carli A., Pane L. & Mariottini G.L. (1998). *Elementi di Ecologia Applicata. Ecotossicologia*. n.6. ECIG Edizioni Culturali Internazionali, ISBN 88-7545-860-X, Genova, Italy.

Cervetto G., Pagano M. & Gaudy R. (1995). Feeding behaviour and migrations in a natural population of the copepod *Acartia tonsa*. *Hydrobiologia*, Vol. 300/301, No. 1 (March 1995), pp. 237-248, ISSN 0018-8158.

Chapman P.M. & Wang F. (2001). Assessing sediment contamination in estuaries. *Environmental Toxicology and Chemistry*, Vol. 20, No. 1 (January 2001), pp. 3-22, ISSN 0730-7268.

Christoffersen K., Hansen B.W., Johansson L.S. & Krog E. (2003). Influence of LAS on marine calanoid copepod population dynamics and potential reproduction. *Aquatic Toxicology*, Vol. 63, No 4 (May 2003), pp. 405-416, ISSN 0166-445X.

Davoren M., Shúilleabháin S.N, O'Halloran J., Hartl M.G.J., Sheehan D., O'Brien N.M., Van Pelt F.N.A.M. & Mothersill C. (2005). A Test Battery Approach for the Ecotoxicological Evaluation of Estuarine Sediments. *Ecotoxicology*, Vol. 14, No. 7 (October 2005), pp. 741-755, ISSN 0963-9292.

Falchier M., Lassus P., Bardouil M., Le Dean L., Truquet P. & Bocquene G. (1981). Sensibilité thermique d'un copépode harpacticoide: *Tigriopus brevicornis* Müller. *Revue des Travaux de l'Institut de Pêches Maritimes*, Vol. 45, No. 1, pp. 141-153, ISSN 0035-2276.

Farabegoli A., Ferrari I., Manzoni C. & Pugnetti E. A. (1989). Prima segnalazione nel Mare Adriatico del copepode calanoide *Acartia tonsa* Dana. *Nova Thalassia*, Vol. 10, No. 1, pp. 207-208.

Faraponova O., Todaro M.A., Onorati F. & Finoia M.G. (2003). Sensibilità sesso ed età specifica di *Tigriopus fulvus* (Copepoda, Harpacticoida) nei confronti di due metalli pesanti (Cadmio e Rame). *Biologia Marina Mediterranea*, Vol. 10, No. 2 (December 2003), pp. 679-681, ISSN 1123-4245.

Forget J., Pavillon J.F., Menasria M.R. & Bocquené G. (1998). Mortality and LC50 values for several stages of the marine copepod *Tigriopus brevicornis* (Müller) exposed to the metals arsenic and cadmium and the pesticides atrazine, carbofuran, dichlorvos, and malathion. *Ecotoxicology and Environmental Safety*, Vol. 40, No. 3 (July 1998), pp. 239-244, ISSN 0147-6513.

Forget J., Beliaeff B. & Bocquené G. (2003). Acetylcholinesterase activity in copepods (*Tigriopus brevicornis*) from the Vilaine River estuary, France, as a biomarker of neurotoxic contaminants. *Aquatic Toxicology*, Vol. 62, No. 3 (February 2003), pp. 195-204, ISSN 0166-445X.

Gaggi C. (1998). Saggi tossicologici di laboratorio. In: *Ecotossicologia*, Vighi M, Bacci E. Eds., pp. 23-39, UTET, ISBN 88-02-05371-5, Torino, Italy.

Gazzetta Ufficiale della Repubblica Italiana (2011). Definizioni delle procedure per il riconoscimento di idoneità dei prodotti assorbenti e disperdenti da impiegare in mare per la bonifica della contaminazione da idrocarburi petroliferi. Supplemento ordinario n. 87, Serie generale – n. 74, 31.3.2011, pp. 35-54.

Giacco E., Greco G., Corrà C., Mariottini G.L., Faimali M. & Pane L. (2006). Toxic response of two Mediterranean crustaceans species to oil dispersants. *Marine Environmental Research*, Vol. 62, supplement, Pollutant Responses in Marine Organisms (PRIMO 13), pp. S54, ISSN 0141-1136.

Hwang D.-S., Lee J.-S., Rhee J.-S., Han J., Lee Y.-M., Kim I.-C., Park G.S., Lee J. & Lee J.-S. (2010). Modulation of p53 gene expression in the intertidal copepod *Tigriopus japonicus* exposed to alkylphenols. *Marine Environmental Research*, Vol. 69, Supplement 1, pp. S77–S80, ISSN 0141-1136.

Invidia M., Sei S. & Gorbi G. (2004). Survival of the copepod *Acartia tonsa* following egg exposure to near anoxia and to sulfide at different pH values. *Marine Ecology Progress Series*, Vol. 276, No. 1, pp. 187-196, ISSN 0171-8630.

IRSA-CNR (1994). *Metodi analitici per le acque*. Poligrafico dello Stato. Quaderno 100, pp. 336–342.

ISO (2005). Water quality – Determination of acute toxicity of marine or estuarine sediment to amphipods. 16712.

Kang S.-W., Seo J., Han J., Lee J.-S. & Jung J. (2011). A comparative study of toxicity identification using *Daphnia magna* and *Tigriopus japonicus*: Implications of establishing effluent discharge limits in Korea. *Marine Pollution Bulletin*, Vol. 63, pp. 370–375, ISSN 0025-326X.

Ki J.-S., Raisuddin S., Lee K.-W., Hwang D.-S., Han J., Rhee J.-S., Kim I.-C., Park H.G., Ryu J.-C. & Lee J.-S. (2009). Gene expression profiling of copper-induced responses in the intertidal copepod *Tigriopus japonicus* using a 6K oligochip microarray. *Aquatic Toxicology*, Vol. 93, No. 4 (July 2009), pp. 177–187, ISSN 0166-445X.

Kim B.-M., Rhee J.-S., Park G.S., Lee J., Lee Y.-M. & Lee J.-S. (2011). Cu/Zn- and Mn-superoxide dismutase (SOD) from the copepod *Tigriopus japonicus*: Molecular cloning and expression in response to environmental pollutants. *Chemosphere*, Vol. 84, No. 10 (September 2011), pp. 1467–1475, ISSN 0045-6535.

Kusk K.O. & Wollenberger L. (2007). Towards an internationally harmonized test method for reproductive and developmental effects of endocrine disrupters in marine copepods. *Ecotoxicology*, Vol. 16, No. 1 (February 2007), pp. 183-195, ISSN 0963-9292.

Kusk K.O, Avdolli M. & Wollenberger L. (2011). Effect of 2,4-dihydroxybenzophenone (BP1) on early life-stage development of the marine copepod *Acartia tonsa* at different temperatures and salinities. *Environmental Toxicology and Chemistry*, Vol. 30, No. 4 (April 2011), pp. 959 966, ISSN 0730-7268.

Kwok K.W.H. & Leung K.M.Y. (2005). Toxicity of antifouling biocides to the intertidal harpacticoid copepod *Tigriopus japonicus* (Crustacea, Copepoda): Effects of temperature and salinity. *Marine Pollution Bulletin*, Vol. 51, pp. 830-837, ISSN 0025-326X.

Kwok K.W.H., Leung K.M.Y., Bao V.W.W. & Lee J.-S. (2008). Copper toxicity in the marine copepod *Tigropus japonicus*: Low variability and high reproducibility of repeated acute and life-cycle tests. *Marine Pollution Bulletin*, Vol. 57, pp. 632–636, ISSN 0025-326X.

Lee Y.-M., Park T.-J., Jung S.-O., Seo J.S., Park H.G., Hagiwara A., Yoon Y.-D. & Lee J.-S. (2006). Cloning and characterization of glutathione S-transferase gene in the intertidal copepod *Tigriopus japonicus* and its expression after exposure to endocrine-disrupting chemicals. *Marine Environmental Research*, Vol. 62, Supplement 1, pp. S219–S223, ISSN 0141-1136.

Lee Y.-M., Lee K.-W., Park H., Park H.G., Raisuddin S., Ahn I.-Y. & Lee J.-S. (2007). Sequence, biochemical characteristics and expression of a novel Sigma-class of glutathione S-transferase from the intertidal copepod, *Tigriopus japonicus* with a possible role in antioxidant defense. *Chemosphere*, Vol. 69, No. 6 (October 2007), pp. 893–902, ISSN 0045-6535.

Lee K.-W., Raisuddin S., Rhee J.-S., Hwang D.-S., Yu I.T., Lee Y.-M., Park H.G. & Lee J.-S. (2008). Expression of glutathione S-transferase (GST) genes in the marine copepod *Tigriopus japonicus* exposed to trace metals. *Aquatic Toxicology*, Vol. 89, No. 3 (September 2008), pp. 158–166, ISSN 0166-445X.

Lera S., Macchia S., Dentone L. & Pellegrini D. (2008). Variations in sensitivity of two populations of *Corophium orientale* (Crustacea: Amphipoda) towards cadmium and sodium laurylsuphate. *Environmental Monitoring and Assessment*, Vol. 136, No. 1-3 (January 2008), pp. 121-127, ISSN 0167-6369.

Liber K, Doig LE & White-Sobey SL. (2011). Toxicity of uranium, molybdenum, nickel, and arsenic to *Hyalella azteca* and *Chironomus dilutus* in water-only and spiked-sediment toxicity tests. *Ecotoxicology and Environmental Safety*, Vol. 74, No. 5 (July 2011), pp. 1171-1179, ISSN 0147-6513.

Macdonald D.D, Ingersoll C.G., Smorong D.E., Sinclair J.A., Lindskoog R., Wang N., Severn C., Gouguet R., Meyer J. & Field J. (2011). Baseline ecological risk assessment of the Calcasieu estuary, Louisiana: part 2. An evaluation of the predictive ability of effects-based sediment-quality guidelines. *Archives of Environmental Contamination and Toxicology*, Vol. 61, No. 1 (July, 2011), pp.14-28, ISSN 0090-4341.

Manfra L., Savorelli F., Migliore L., Magaletti E. & Cicero A.M. (2009). Saggio di tossicità a 14 giorni con *Artemia franciscana*: validazione del metodo. *Biologia Marina Mediterranea*, Vol. 14, No. 2, pp. 15-18, ISSN 1123-4245.

Mann R.M., Hyne R.V. & Ascheri L.M. (2011). Foraging, feeding, and reproduction on silica substrate: Increased waterborne zinc toxicity to the estuarine epibenthic amphipod *Melita plumulosa*. *Environmental Toxicology and Chemistry*, Vol. 30, No. 7 (July, 2011), pp. 1649-1658, ISSN 0730-7268.

Medina M., Barata C., Telfer T. & Baird D.J. (2002). Age- and sex-related variation in sensitivity to the pyrethroid cypermethrin in the marine copepod *Acartia tonsa* Dana. *Archives of Environmental Contamination and Toxicology*, Vol. 42, No. 1 (January 2002), pp. 17-22, ISSN 0090-4341.

Mille G., Munoz D., Jacquot F., Rivet L. & Bertrand J. C. (1998). The Amoco CadizOil spill: Evolution of petroleum hydrocarbons in the Ile Grande salt marshes (Brittany) after a 13-year period. *Estuarine, Coastal and Shelf Science*, Vol. 47, No. 5 (November 1998), pp. 547-559, ISSN 0272-7714.

Müller H.G. (1980). Experiences with test systems using *Daphnia magna*. *Ecotoxicology and Environmental Safety*, Vol. 4, No. 1 (March 1980), pp. 21-25, ISSN 0147-6513.

OECD (2004). *Daphnia* sp. Acute Immobilisation Test. OECD Guidelines for the Testing of Chemicals / Section 2: Effects on Biotic Systems. Test No. 202, pp. 1-12.

OECD (2008). *Daphnia magna* Reproduction Test. OECD Guidelines for the Testing of Chemicals / Section 2: Effects on Biotic Systems. Test No. 211, pp. 1-23.

Onorati F. & Volpi Ghirardini A. (2001). Informazioni fornite dalle diverse matrici da testare con i saggi biologici: applicabilità di *Vibrio fischeri*. *Biologia Marina Mediterranea*, Vol. 8, No. 2, pp. 31-40, ISSN 1123-4245.

OSPAR (1995). PARCOM Protocols on methods for the testing of chemicals used in the offshore oil industry. OSPAR Commission, ISBN 0946956448, pp. 1-35.

Pane L., De Nuccio L., Pruzzo C. & Carli A. (2000). Adhesion of bacteria and diatoms to the exoskeleton of the harpacticoid copepod *Tigriopus fulvus* in culture: electron and epifluorescent microscope study. *Journal of Biological Research – Bollettino della Società Italiana di Biologia Sperimentale*, Vol. 76, No. 5-6 (May-June 2000), pp. 37-43, ISSN 0037-8771.

Pane L., De Nuccio L. & Franceschi E., (2003). Contenuto energetico del copepode *Tigriopus fulvus* (Fischer 1860): applicazione della DSC (Differential Scanning Calorimetry). *Biologia Marina Mediterranea*, Vol. 10, No. 2 (December 2003), pp. 593-596, ISSN 1123-4245.

Pane L., Giacco E. & Mariottini G.L. (2006a). Utilizzo di *Tigriopus fulvus* (Copepoda: Harpacticoida) in ecotossicologia. Saggi con disperdenti e tensioattivi. Atti XXXVII Congresso SIBM, Grosseto, 5-10 giugno 2006, *Biologia Marina Mediterranea*, Vol. 13, No. 2 (May 2006), pp. 348-349, ISSN 1123-4245.

Pane L., Giacco E. & Mariottini G.L. (2006b). Acute and chronic heavy metal bioassay on *Tigriopus fulvus* Fischer (Copepoda: Harpacticoida). *Marine Environmental Research*, Vol. 62, supplement, Pollutant Responses in Marine Organisms (PRIMO 13), pp. S95, ISSN 0141-1136.

Pane L., Giacco E. & Mariottini G.L. (2007a). Uso di *Tigriopus fulvus* (Copepoda: Harpacticoida) nella valutazione del rischio ecotossicologico in ambiente marino. *Biologia Marina Mediterranea*, Vol. 14, No. 1 (April 2008), pp. 186-188, ISSN 1123-4245.

Pane L., Giacco E. & Mariottini G.L. (2007b). Effect of surfactants on the reproduction of *Tigriopus fulvus* Fischer. *Experimental Biology Reports*, Vol. 1, No. 1 (July 2008), pp. 77-88, ISBN 978-88-491-3092-8.

Pane L., Giacco E., Corrà C., Greco G., Mariottini G.L., Varisco F. & Faimali M. (2008a). Ecotoxicological evaluation of harbour sediments using marine organisms. *Journal of Soils and Sediments*, Vol. 8, No. 2, pp. 74-79, ISSN 1439-0108.

Pane L., Mariottini G.L., Lodi A. & Giacco E. (2008b). Effects of heavy metals on laboratory reared *Tigriopus fulvus* Fischer (Copepoda: Harpacticoida). In: *"Heavy Metal Pollution"* (Samuel E. Brown and William C. Welton Eds.), Nova Science Publishers Inc., ISBN-13 978-1-60456-899-8, ISBN-10 1-60456-899-2, Hauppauge NY. Chapter 6, 157-165.

Pane L., Giacco E. & Mariottini G.L. (2009). Utilizzo del copepode *Tigriopus fulvus* in studi tossicologici alternativi. In: *Innovazione chimica per l'applicazione del REACH*, Campanella L., Tapparo A., De Gennaro G., Barbieri P., Passarini F., Mazzone A. (Eds.), pp. (43-45), Società Chimica Italiana, Milano, Italy.

Pane L. & Mariottini G.L. (2009). Uso di colture cellulari di pesce in ecotossicologia. In: *Innovazione chimica per l'applicazione del REACH*, Campanella L., Tapparo A., De Gennaro G., Barbieri P., Passarini F., Mazzone A. (Eds.), pp. (45-47), Società Chimica Italiana, Milano, Italy.

Pane L. & Mariottini G.L. (2010). Characteristics of the rocky littoral system. Biological and ecological aspects. In: *Rock Chemistry* , Basilio Macias and Fidel Guajardo Editors, pp. 121-130, Nova Science Publishers, Inc., ISBN 978-1-60876-563-8, Hauppauge NY.

Paoletti R., Nicosia S., Clementi F. & Fumagalli G. (1998). *Ecotossicologia. Trattato di farmacologia e terapia*, Vighi M., Bacci E. (Eds.). UTET, ISBN 88-02-05371-5, Torino, Italy.

Peters C. & Ahlf W. (2005). Reproduction of the estuarine and marine amphipod *Corophium volutator* (Pallas) in laboratory for toxicity testing. *Chemosphere*, Vol. 59, No. 4 (April 2005), pp. 525-536, ISSN 0045-6535.

Persoone G. & Janssen C.R. (1998). Freshwater invertebrate toxicity tests, In: *Handbook of Ecotoxicology*, Peter Calow (Ed.), pp. (51-65), Blackwell Science, ISBN 978-0-632-04933-2, Oxford, UK.

Rhee J.-S., Raisuddin S., Lee K.-W., Seo J.S., Ki J.-S., Kim I.-C., Park H.G. & Lee J.-S. (2009). Heat shock protein (Hsp) gene responses of the intertidal copepod *Tigriopus japonicus* to environmental toxicants. *Comparative Biochemistry and Physiology, Part C*, Vol. 149, No. 1 (Januaty 2009), pp. 104–112, ISSN 1532-0456.

Rose M. 1933. *Faune de France. 26, Copépodes pélagiques*, Paul Lechevalier, Paris, France.

Sei S., Rossetti G., Villa F. & Ferrari I. (1996). Zooplankton variability related to environmental changes in a eutrophic coastal lagoon in the Po Delta. *Hydrobiologia*, Vol. 329, No. 1-3, pp. 45-55, ISSN 0018-8158.

Shaw I.C. & Chadwick J. (1995). Ecotoxicity Testing. *Toxicology & Ecotoxicology News*, Vol. 2, No. 3, pp. 80-85, ISSN 1350-4592.

Solbé J.F. De L.G. (1998). Freshwater fish. In : *Handbook of Ecotoxicology*, Calow P. Ed., pp. 66-82, Blackwell Science, ISBN 978-0-632-04933-2, Oxford, UK.

Strom D., Simpson S.L., Batley G.E. & Jolley D.F. (2011). The influence of sediment particle size and organic carbon on toxicity of copper to benthic invertebrates in oxic/suboxic surface sediments. *Environmental Toxicology and Chemistry*, Vol. 30, No. 7 (July 2011), pp. 1599-1610, ISSN 0730-7268.

Sverdrup L.E., Fürst C.S., Weideborg M., Vik E.A. & Stenersen J. (2002). Relative sensitivity of one freshwater and two marine acute toxicity tests as determined by testing 30 offshore E & P chemicals. *Chemosphere*, Vol. 46, No. 2 (January 2002), pp. 311-318, ISSN 0045-6535.

Todaro M.A., Faraponova O., Onorati F., Pellegrini D. & Tongiorgi P. (2001). *Tigriopus fulvus* (Copepoda, Harpacticoda) una possible specie-target nella valutazione della tossicità dei fanghi portuali: ciclo vitale e prove tossicologiche preliminari. *Biologia Marina Mediterranea*, Vol. 8, No. 1, pp. 896-872, ISSN 1123-4245.

Weideborg M., Vik E.A., Øfkord G.D. & Kjønnø O. (1997). Comparison of three marine screening tests and four Oslo and Paris Commission procedures to evaluate toxicity of offshore chemicals. *Environmental Toxicology and Chemistry*, Vol. 16, No. 2 (February 1997), pp. 384-389, ISSN 0730-7268.

Widdows J. (1998). Marine and estuarine invertebrate toxicity tests, In: *Handbook of Ecotoxicology*, Peter Calow (Ed.), pp. (145-166) Blackwell Science, ISBN 978-0-632-04933-2, Oxford, UK.

Wollenberger L., Dinan L. & Breitholtz M. (2005). Brominated flame retardants: activities in a crustacean development test and in an ecdysteroid screening assay. *Environmental Toxicology and Chemistry*, Vol. 24, No. 2 (February 2005), pp. 400-407, ISSN 0730-7268.

Zanders I. P. & Rojas W. E. (1992). Cadmium accumulation, LC50 and oxygen consumption in the tropical marine amphipod *Elasmopus rapax*. *Marine Biology*, Vol. 113, No. 3 (July 1992), pp. 409-413, ISSN 0025-3162.

5

Alternative Biotest on *Artemia franciscana*

Petr Dvorak[1], Katarina Benova[2] and Jiri Vitek[1]
[1]University of Veterinary and Pharmaceutical Sciences
[2]University of Veterinary Medicine and Pharmacy
[1]Czech Republic
[2]Slovak Republic

1. Introduction

Recent toxicology, in accordance with recommendations from the European Council, has demanded decrease in the number of vertebrates used in toxicology testing and their partial replacement with invertebrate animals, plants or even organ, tissue, or cell cultures. During the last 50 years various invertebrate species have been tested for their sensitivity to many chemical or physical agents to prove their possible use for pre-screening tests. To the most valuable organisms available for ecotoxicity testing belong crustaceans of the *Artemia* genus, commonly known as brine shrimps.

2. Characterisation of *Artemia franciscana*

The taxonomic status of the *Artemia* genus is as follows (Martin & Davis, 2001):
Subphylum: Crustacea Brünnich, 1772
Class: Branchiopoda Latreille, 1817
Subclass: Sarsostraca Tasch, 1969
Order: Anostraca Sars, 1867
Family: Artemiidae Grochowski, 1896
Genus: *Artemia* Leach, 1819.
To this genus belong the following species:

A. salina, monica, urmiana, franciscana, persimilis, sinica, tibetiana, sp. Pilla & Beardmore 1994, and parthenogenetic population(s) of Europe, Africa, Asia, and Australia. In this report we use *A. franciscana* Kellogg 1906, distributed in America, Caribbean, and Pacific islands.

Populations of the *Artemia* genus are widely distributed in all continents except for Antarctica. Species of this genus inhabit more than 500 salt lakes, but not seas, of temperate, subtropical, and tropical zones. They are very well adapted to high salinity waters (up to 70 g.L⁻¹, but can survive even at 250 g.L⁻¹, Ruppert & Barnes, 1994) with fairly low diversity of living organisms and absence of predators or competitive species. In these environments the evolution of *Artemia* species is favoured by the abundance of microorganisms such as bacteria, protozoa and algae that are the basis of the *Artemia* diet (Amat, 1985).

Brine shrimps come in many colours - from white to pink, shadow, or green. The different colours probably result from specific diets and environmental conditions. Females can reach

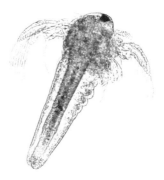

Fig. 1. Nauplius of *A. franciscana*.

the size of 30 mm (most often 12 - 18 mm), males are smaller. Their body is divided into three parts: head, thorax, and abdomen. On the head there is a pair of stalked, lateral, compound eyes and a single, median, unstalked naupliar eye, and two pairs of antennae. The latter are sexually dimorphic. Those of the adult males are modified to form a clasping organ to hold the female during copulation. The female antennae are smaller but much thicker and have a sensorial function. The remainder of the body consists of the segmented thorax, consisted of 11 segments, and posterior abdomen. Each thoracic segment bears a ventral pair of leaf-like appendages, known as phyllopods, used for swimming, respiration, and feeding. Finally, the abdomen consists of 6 segments and a telson – the posterior end of the body. The abdomen of females carries a bunch of spherical-like eggs (cca 200 u in diameter). Their colour varies from creamy to almost blackish brown (Anderson, 1967; Benesch, 1969; Hertel, 1980).

The brine shrimp larva – nauplius is pink or rather auburn, its size about 0.4 mm. Its body consists of a head and short thorax (Fig. 1). On the head there is a dark, red or black, median naupliar eye and two pairs of antennae. The second pair is used for swimming and feeding, while the first pair is a sensory organ.

Artemia franciscana is resistant to high osmotic stress of the hypersaline environments. Its nauplii drink water and secret Na^+ and Cl^- ions. The adults ingest water by mouth and anus. The capability to ingest water, containing bacteria and debris as well, is developed in the 2nd instar stage (Kikuchi, 1971). The larvae hatch usually after 20 - 48 hrs of embryonic development and reach their terminal size after 8 - 10 days, during which they undergo about 17 molts (Gilchrist, 1960).

The life span of *A. franciscana* varies from 2 to 4 months in dependence on salinity and temperature (Browne et al., 1991). Reproduction of the genus *Artemia* may proceed in two modalities: sexual or parthenogenetic. Both, sexual and parthenogenetic populations occur all over the world except for Americas where only sexual populations have been reported (Browne, 1992). Coexistence of both sexual and parthenogenetic strains has been recorded in various habitats; however, partial overlapping in space and/or time may occur. The parthenogenetic reproduction results in unisexual, female populations. While the bisexual specimens have stable number of chromosomes (2n = 42), the parthenogenetic populations may be diploid, triploid, tetraploid, or even pentaploid (Hentschel, 1968).

Females after insemination produce eggs that start to develop immediately after laying. But, under unfavourable conditions dormant stages, known as cysts, are produced. Their metabolism is inhibited and they can survive, even in extreme conditions, for dozens of years. In the cyst there is an embryo in the stage of gastrula, enwrapped with a hard outer membrane. In natural habitats the cysts gather on the water surface, and then drift ashore where they survive the unfavourable season. When the cysts occur in salt water their metabolic activity is again restored and in 20 hrs hatches the umbrella stage that quickly develops to a free swimming nauplius (Browne et al., 1991).

Artemia cysts are produced mainly in the USA, Australia, China, or Saudi Arabia but other countries are also involved. The recent annual yield of the cysts is about 2 000 t. They are produced for the aquaculture or aquarium practice as food for tropical fish. One of the most important sources of the cysts is the Great Salt Lake in Utah, USA. In the northern part (Gunnison Bay) *Artemia salina* cysts are produced in 16 oz. (454 g) cans, while in the southern part (Gilbert Bay) *Artemia franciscana* is produced and packed in 15 oz. (425 g) cans. The latter cysts are more delicate (more than 300 000 specimens per 1 g). The best quality products are sold as the Premium class, and this quality was used in our experiments ("Maxima brine shrimp eggs" produced by the Sanders firm in Utah).

3. Alternative methods

Alternative methods are as follows:

- biotests on plants (e.g. mustard roots, soya, or rice; Horowitz, 1970; Kratky & Warren, 1971) or algae (e.g. *Selenastrum capricornutum, Chlorella kesssleri, or Chlamydomonas reinhardtii*; Fouradzieva et al., 1995);
- biotests on invertebrates (e.g. *Daphnia magna, Tetrahymena piriformis, Asellus aquaticus*, genus *Tubifex*, or flatworms; Balls et al., 1992);
- biotests on vertebrates in early stages of development, before a nervous system is developed and the specimens do not feel any pain (Bagley et al., 1994);
- in vitro methods, i.e., cell, tissue, or organ cultures (Fentem & Balls, 1993), and
- mathematical and computer simulations (Pazourek, 1992).

The methods mentioned above have some disadvantages. Most of them are time consuming, require skilled workers, and often are expensive. These disadvantages may be overcome by the alternative microbiotests, in which the effect of dissolved agents on unicellular or small multicellular organisms is evaluated. For such tests are convenient various simple organisms, such as bacteria, fungi, algae, protozoa, or invertebrates (Blaise, 1991).

In the Multicenter Evaluation of In Vitro Toxicity (MEIC) program the special list of chemical agents have been proved in four standardized tests of the acute toxicity realized on the following species: *Artemia franciscana, Streptocephalus proboscideus, Brachionus calyciflorus,* and *Brachionus plicatilis*. The mortality and toxic effects expressed as $LC_{50/24}$ (i.s., the concentration of an agent at which 50 per cent of the tested animals are dead after 24 hrs) were chosen as criteria of the toxicity. Very good correlations of results among the different testing systems have been found. Furthermore, positive correlations between the tests on lower organisms and conventional tests on rats have also been achieved (Calleja & Persoone, 1992).

The "toxkit" tests are based on dormant stages – cysts or ephippia - that hatch up to 24 hrs before the start of a test. Their advantage is particularly the elimination of time and space consuming laboratory maintenance of the test organisms. Commercially available are ROTOXKIT F, ROTOXKIT M, THAMNOTOXKIT F, ARTOXKIT M, etc.

3.1 Alternative biotests on *Artemia* species

Suitability of the *Artemia* species for the toxicity studies was recognized 80 years ago (Boone, 1931). The first bioassay on *Artemia salina* was offered by Michael et al. (1956). Twenty four years later the standardized acute toxicity bioassay - Artoxkit M (Microbiotests, Inc., Mariakerke /Gent/ - Belgium) was developed (Vanhaecke et al., 1980). The reliability and validity of this commercially available test have been confirmed by a large international study (Vanhaecke & Persoone, 1981). Later on, Solis et al. (1993) developed the Artemia Microwell Cytotoxicity Assay.

Various modifications of the biotests on *Artemia* species have been used for the acute or rarely chronic toxicity testing of a large number of inorganic substances: such as cadmium (Hadjispyrou et al., 2001; Sarabia et al., 1998a, 2002, 2006; Brix et al., 2006), mercury (Sarabia et al., 1998b), chromium (Hadjispyrou et al., 2001), stannum (Hadjispyrou et al., 2001), zinc (Brix et al., 2006), copper (Browne, 1980, Brix et al., 2006), arsenic (Brix et al., 2003), potassium permanganate, potassium bichromate, and silver nitrate (see Boone, 1931), phenolic compounds (Guerra, 2001), and trace elements (Petruci et al., 1995). From the organic substances have been tested: organic solvents (Barahona-Gomariz et al., 1994), acrylonitrile (Tong et al., 1996), antifouling agents (Okamura et al., 2000), oil dispersants (Zillioux, et al., 1973), phorbol esters (Kinghorn et al., 1977), phthalates (Van Wezel, et al., 2000), carbamates (Barahona & Sánchez-Fortún, 1998), atropine (Barahona & Sánchez-Fortún, 1998), anesthetics (Robinson et al., 1965), antihelmintics (Oliveira-Filho & Paumgartten, 2000), herbicides, insecticides, pesticides (Varó et al., 1997, 2002), mycotoxins (Schmidt, 1985; Panigrahi, 1993; Hlywka et al., 1997), pharmaceuticals (Touraki et al., 1999, Parra et al., 2001), pollutants (Knulst & Sodergren, 1994), opiates (Richter & Goldstein, 1970), various plant extracts (Cáceres et al., 1998), or toxins (Granade et al. 1976; Vezie et al., 1996; Beattie et al., 2003). The tests on the genus *Artemia* have also been used to specify biological effects of some physical factors, such as ionizing radiation (Grosch & Erdman, 1955; Easter & Hutchinson, 1961), radionuclides (Boroughs et al., 1958), or UV (Dattilo et al., 2005). In the project Biostack carried out on Apollo 16 the effects of cosmic irradiation on cysts of *Artemia franciscana* were studied (Ruther et al., 1974; Graul et al., 1975; Heinrich, 1977).

3.2 Advantages and disadvantages of the *Artemia* species for toxicity test

The *Artemia* species have been found convenient for various short- or long-term toxicity testing. In spite of this fact, several criticisms against their suitability for such purpose have been published (Persoone & Wells, 1987; Nunes et al., 2006). The most important of them is the lower sensitivity of the *Artemia* species to several chemical or physical agents in comparison to the other invertebrate test organisms (Sorgeloos et al., 1978; Song and Brown, 1998, Okamura et al., 2000; Guerra, 2001; Nalecz-Jawecki et al., 2003; George-Ares, et al., 2003; Mayorga et al., 2010). The second disadvantage is a decreased solubility of some chemical substances in saline or sea medium (e.g. Mayorga et al., 2010), however, this problem may be overcome by using convenient co-solvents (see bellow).

In general, the reliability of results of the *Artemia* tests may be affected by various conditions of a test, such as temperature, pH, chemical composition of the medium, oxygen, photoperiod, nutrients, some population effects, type of sexual reproduction, etc. (Soares, et al., 1992). For example, George-Ares et al. (2003) reported dependence of the *Artemia* test on the concentration and composition of medium, or on the age of nauplii. Some populations of *Artemia* species may consist of strains with different reproduction strategies (sexual versus parthenogenetic reproduction) and different sensitivity to tested agents. But, Triantaphyllidis et al. (1994) suggested a simple method to separate nauplii of bisexual and parthenogenetic strains by hatching at different temperatures, moreover specific strains may be distinguished by DNA-analysis (Abatzopoulos et al., 1997). Of course, the effects of almost all test factors mentioned above may be easily overcome by the strict standardization of test conditions. An important disadvantage of all alternative tests is their unsuitability to test the chemical agents that require metabolic activation in mammals.

On the other hand, the *Artemia* alternative tests offer many advantages to favour them as convenient for the standardized testing in ecotoxicology: high adaptability to variety of testing conditions, high fecundity, bisexual versus parthenogenetic reproduction strategies, small body size, varied nutrient resources, high hatchability, simple availability, and low cost of the tests. High sensitivity of the *Artemia* specimens to some chemical agents has also been reported. For example, Oliveira-Filho and Paumgartten (2000) found the higher sensitivity of *Artemia* to niclosamide in comparison with *Daphnia similis* or *Ceriodaphnia dubia*. Hlywka et al. (1997) have shown similar sensitivities to the mycotoxin fumonisin B1 in the *Artemia* test and the chicken embryo screening test. And Parra et al. (2001) compared the sensitivity of the acute toxicity *Artemia* test of several plant extracts with corresponding tests on mice and found significant correlations. Undoubtedly, the *Artemia* test is a suitable, sufficiently accurate, simple, and inexpensive alternative to pre-screening chemical toxicity with mammals. Of course, all results derived from the *Artemia* or any other invertebrate test have to be validated by bioassays on mammals.

Our test is based on the cysts produced for purposes of the aquaculture and aquarium practice. The test was established in 1992 (Dvorak, 1995), especially for the extensive dynamic studies including simultaneous treatments with two agents, or possibly of a radiation and a chemical agent. The total expenses of our tests are lower than those of the commercial toxkits.

4. Methods

4.1 Hatching of cysts

Cysts are hatched in water of the following composition (Table 1). The total concentration of salts is 4.7%. In the following text this water is specified as the "sea water".

In water of this quality the brine shrimps mature in 37 days and start their reproduction, providing they are fed with a convenient diet, and the sea water is changed every third day. The hatching proceeds at temperature of 25 °C and the first larvae occur after 24 hrs. During the hatching process the sea water is aerated by a membrane compressor.

salt (per analysis)	$g.L^{-1}$
NaCl	23.900
$MgCl_2 . 6H_2O$	10.830
$CaCl_2 . 6H_2O$	2.250
KCl	0.680
$Na_2SO_4 . 10 H_2O$	9.060
$NaHCO_3$	0.200
$SrCl_2 . 6H_2O$	0.040
KBr	0.099
H_3BO_3	0.027

Table 1. Composition of hatching water.

4.2 Solubility of chemical agents

Solubility of various chemical agents in 4.7% sea water is often decreased. Consequently, in our pharmacological studies the concentration of sea water is reduced to 0.9% (i.e. the concentration of the blood salts). But, in this low concentration of salt water *A. franciscana* does not consume glucose; consequently, in such low concentration of medium this sugar cannot be used to prolong the test.

The solubility of some low soluble chemical agents may be improved by specific co-solvents. For example, increased solubility of some insoluble purine inhibitors of cyclin-dependent kinases may be achieved by the non-ionic tensides: polysorbate 80 and poloxamer Pluronic F68.

The co-solvent is a non-water solvent that can be mixed with water and the resulting mixture has increased capability to solve some chemical compounds. For example, dimethylsulfoxide (DMSO) is used as solvent and co-solvent for its ability to solve the most of organic or inorganic chemical compounds, as well as an enhancer of some medicines into skin. It is a colourless liquid, hygroscopic and miscible with water and many other organic solvents (Rowe et al., 2006). DMSO is included in some veterinary medicines. In medicaments used in human medicine it is used only rarely for some undesirable effects. The analgetic, antiflogistic, vasodilatative, myorelaxative, and antiviral effects of DMSO have been reported (Jacob & Herschler, 1986; Rowe et al., 2006). The systemic toxicity of this drug in vivo is rather low (Rowe et al., 2006).

The tweens are used in the pharmaceutical, cosmetics or food industries. Polysorbate 80 (Tween 80) is the tenside widely used in pharmaceuticals as helping agents for the preparation of oral or parenteral suspensions. In parenteral medicines the content of this agent must not exceed the concentration in which it causes a hemolysis of erythrocytes (Rowe et al., 2006). It is an oil-like, yellowish but clear liquid with a specific odour and rather bitter taste. This substance is miscible with water or ethylacetate, but insoluble in fatty oils or a paraffine liquid. The pH value of a 5% water solution varies from 6.0 to 8.0. Chemically it is a polyoxyethylensorbitanmonooleate and it consists of the partial esters of sorbitol and its anhydrides, copolymerized with cca 20 moles of ethylenoxide per mol of sorbitol and sorbitol anhydrides with various fatty acids, mainly the oleic acid. The toxicity of polysorbate 80 is rather low – the acute toxicity LD_{50} in mice treated perorally is 25 $g.kg^{-1}$

(Rowe et al., 2006). We used polysorbate 80 produced by the Jan Kulich firm (Hradec Kralove, Czech Republic) applied in mixture with DMSO. Concentration of the stock solution of polysorbate 80 was 200 g.L^{-1}. In our experiments we combined the concentrations 10.0 g.L^{-1} of polysorbate 80 and 5.0 g.L^{-1} of DMSO.

Poloxamers are non-ionic agents used in pharmaceuticals as emulgators, sufractants, wetting agents, or solubilisers. In pharmaceuticals, they are widely used as helping agents for various medications. These agents are non-toxic, non-irritable and are not metabolised in the living organisms. For their inability to cause a hemolysis (Rowe et al., 2006) they are used in various parenteral medicaments. Poloxamers are commercially produced under the names of Lutrol® or Pluronic® (e.g. commercial name of the Poloxamer 188 used in this study is Pluronic F68). The acute toxicity of these agents applied in mice is 15 g.kg^{-1}, if applied perorally, or 1 g.kg^{-1}, when applied parenteraly (Rowe et al., 2006). In our experiments we used a concentration of 10.0 g.L^{-1} applied with DMSO.

4.3 Treatment with polychlorinated biphenyls and ionizing radiation

Delor 103 is one of the polychlorinated biphenyls (PCB's). These compounds produce colloidal solutions. The initial delor 103 colloidal solution in salt water was obtained by three-day agitation. The excessive undissolved delor 103 was then removed. For the treatment we used the concentration of 4.5 ng.L^{-1}. This final concentration was detected by the capillary gas column chromatography analysis (41 peaks identified; from dichloride to pentachloride derivatives). The Kovats index was used as a method of evaluation.

As source of ionizing radiation we used the beta emitter strontium 89 in solution with the volume activity of 33 kBq.L^{-1}. The isotope was supplied by the Amersham Comp. as strontium chloride dissolved in water. The manufacturer guarantees specific strontium activity of 1.85 - 7.40 GBq.g^{-1} and purity $< 0.5\%$ ^{85}Sr $< 0.1\%$ ^{90}Sr, with pH within the 5.0 - 9.0 range. The final activity used in experiments was obtained by re-calculation of the original activity to the reference date. Potassium dichromate $K_2Cr_2O_7$ of analytical grade was used in the concentration of 5 mg.L^{-1} and cadmium chloride $CdCl_2 . 2.5H_2O$ in the final concentration of 20 mg.L^{-1}.

4.4 Subacute toxicity

Ten freshly hatched nauplii are placed into a polystyrene Petri dish (diameter 60 mm) by a thin plastic Pasteur pipette. The total volume of salt water is adjusted to 9 ml per dish. All the agents tested are dissolved in sea water, always in a concentration ten times higher than that finally required for a treatment. Consequently, to a dish with 9 ml of the standard sea water 1 ml of the tenfold concentrated stock solution is supplemented (in case of the control dishes 1 ml of the standard salt water). If the simultaneous treatment of two agents is tested, the original volume of sea water with specimens per dish is 8 ml and then each agent is supplemented in 1 ml of its stock solution.

The biotest proceeds in darkness, at temperature of 20 ± 0.5 °C, in covered dishes, and without aeration. The specimens are not fed, and consequently, under these conditions they start to die of starvation after 120 hrs. When the temperature is increased to 24 °C the lifespan of unfed nauplii is shortened to about 96 hrs.

For every experimental combination five Petri dishes (50 specimens in total) are used. Alive specimens are counted after 24, 48, 72, 96, or 120 hrs (in case of prolonged tests). The dead nauplii are not removed but their presence has not any deleterious effect on the final results of the biotest. If more than 10% of the experimental specimens died in the control group, the exposure was discarded. The evaluation of results of an experimental series should be always performed by one person.

As dead we consider the specimens that do not move even after the stimulation by movement of water caused by rotation of the dish. The evaluation is carried out under a microscope or magnifying glass. To express results of such a test, two terms are, generally used: mortality and lethality. The first means the percentage of dead specimens from the total number of originally healthy specimens. On the other hand, lethality means the percentage of dead specimens from all ill specimens. We use the latter term because, in fact, all specimens exposed to the agents tested at first become ill and only then some of them die.

4.5 Long term toxicity

The prolongation of life span of nauplii in biotests may be achieved by feeding. However, utilisation of various artificial diets, algae or yeast is always complicated with the contamination with some undesired chemical substances or metabolites. Hence, we prolong the *Artemia* test by the treatment with 3% solution of glucose that is used by the specimens as a source of energy. The other parameters of prolonged tests correspond to those of the standard test. The evaluation of results is carried out in steps of 24 hrs for 10 days (Dvorak et al., 2005).

4.6 Expression of concentrations

Concentrations of agents may be expressed in toxicology in mmol.L^{-1} or mg.L^{-1} (in some papers is used ppm unit, but it is not included in the International System of Units). The first method is used to compare different chemical compounds which toxicity depends on only part of the molecule, such as cations of metals, or molecules accompanied with bound molecules of water. In these cases the concentration is expressed only for the active part of the molecule (e.g. mmol $Cd^{2+}.L^{-1}$). This expression accentuates rather more the chemical properties of the molecule than its biological effects. Actually, a biological effect often depends on physical properties of the agent, particularly on its solubility and absorption. Consequently, we prefer the expression of concentrations in units of weight, providing that the precise chemical composition of the substance is included. For this reason we express the drug concentrations in our experiments in mg.L^{-1}.

4.7 Evaluation of results

All 50 specimens (i.e., 5 Petri dishes with 10 specimens each) of one experimental combination are evaluated as a whole. Each specimen is judged as alive or dead (criterion see above). Significance of results is calculated according to Hayes (1991). The lethality is expressed in percentage of all specimens used. Results are displayed in the form of 3D charts – concentrations versus time of treatment.

4.8 Validity of results

The principle validity criterion of results is the mortality in control dishes lower than 10%. This criterion is generally used in the *Artemia*, as well as, in *Dafnia* toxicity tests. Because the specimens in our experimental system are not fed and starve, it is sometimes difficult to keep this criterion at the exposures higher than 72 hrs. In this case, we terminate the experiments at this exposure, in spite of the fact that in the exposure of 96 hrs the nauplii are the most sensitive to some toxic agents and difference between the treated and control group is the highest. In the prolonged experiments (120 hrs or more) in medium supplemented with glucose (see above) we use the higher criterion of mortality (20%). The glucose is probably not sufficient to secure the optimal development of the experimental specimens. Consequently, we generally finish experiments when the mortality of the control group exceeds 20%.

5. Results and discussion

5.1 Simultaneous treatment with ^{89}Sr and low concentrations of cadmium, chromium, and delor 103

For principal information about the treatment with polychlorinated biphenyls and ionizing radiation see 4.3. Results are summarized in Fig. 2. Neither the treatment with delor 103 or ^{89}Sr per se, nor the simultaneous treatment with the both agents did not affect survival of the experimental specimens (results of the separate treatments are not included in figure, simultaneous treatment see 'PCB + Strontium 89' in Fig. 2). On the contrary, potassium dichromate increased the lethality up to 27% (at 72 hrs). The simultaneous treatments with two agents (cadmium + potassium dichromate) or with all four agents altogether (cadmium + potassium dichromate + delor 130 + ^{89}Sr) resulted in the expressive increase in lethality of the experimental specimens.

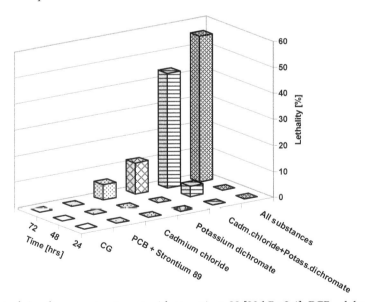

Fig. 2. Effect of simultaneous treatment with strontium 89 [33 kBq.L^{-1}], PCB - delor 103 [4.5 ng.L^{-1}], cadmium chloride (CdCl$_2$. 2H$_2$O) [Cadm.chloride; 20 mg.L^{-1}], and potassium dichromate [Potass.dichromate; 5 mg.L^{-1}] on lethality of A. *franciscana* ; CG – control group (no agents).

Isotope ^{89}Sr is a beta emitter; consequently, it is impossible to satisfactorily convert its activity to a dose the experimental specimens actually receive during the exposure. For this reason, the strontium effects are given in the volume activity units of kBq.L[-1]. The hexavalent chromium can damage DNA, decrease its synthesis and enhance the oxidative processes in cells. The analogous effects are induced by the ionizing radiation, as well.

Both agents - strontium 89 or delor 103 - attack the membrane integrity, the result of which may be the increased penetration of potassium dichromate or cadmium chloride into cells. Cadmium induces production of metallothioneins (e.g. Huska et al., 2008) that express, among others, the radioprotective effects (Benova et al., 2006).

This study demonstrated the suitability of the *Artemia* test to evaluate effects of rather complex experiments with simultaneous treatments of several chemical and/or physical agents.

5.2 Changes in morphology of *Artemia* specimens during treatment with gamma rays or inhibitors of cyclin-dependent kinases

In our previous paper the lethality of *A. franciscana* after irradiation with the ionizing radiation was studied. The LD_{50} value was estimated 96 hrs after the irradiation with 600 - 700 Gy (Dvorak & Benova, 2002). This result is in accord with the phylogenetic position of this species.

In the following experimental series the freshly hatched nauplii were irradiated by the gamma rays (^{60}Co) with 100, 250, 500, or 1000 Gy (dose rate of 2.7 kGy.h[-1]). At the time of 72 or 96 hrs after the irradiation the specimens were killed and fixed with formaldehyde. The morphological changes were determined and documented by microphotography.

During the standard development of the control group we observed segmentation of the thoracal part and formation of appendages. The development of those structures in the specimens irradiated with 100 Gy (96 hrs after the irradiation) was comparable with control specimens. But after the irradiation with 250 Gy the segmentation was less apparent, and at the highest doses (500 or 1000 Gy) it was not observed at all.

Another morphological change observed after the irradiation was an atypical development of the intestine epithelium. In control specimens the ratio of the height of epithelium to the diameter of intestine lumen was 1 : 1.2. After irradiation the ratio changed: with 100 Gy to 1 : 1.3, with 250 Gy to 1 : 1.5, and even with 500 Gy to 1 : 1.8. When the doses increased to 1000 Gy the intestine epithelium was undistinguishable. The high sensitivity of intestine epithelium to irradiation corresponds with high sensitivity of this tissue in vertebrates caused by the high mitotic activity of intestine cells. Consequently, the effects of irradiation on the intestine epithelium in the *Artemia* species were consistent with the analogous response in vertebrates.

We also looked for some morphological changes caused by the inhibitors of the cyclin-dependent kinases – olomoucin or roscovitin to compare them with effects of the ionizing radiation. Both agents, in the concentration of 100 mg.L[-1], caused only slight changes in the intestine epithelium of nauplii stages of *A. franciscana*, but they did not affect the segmentation of thorax and further development of appendages. Also the length or morphology of the body were not affected by these drugs. In the concentration of 50 mg.L[-1] no effects on the intestine epithelium were apparent.

5.3 Toxicity of newly synthesized inhibitors of cyclin-dependent kinases

The synthetic inhibitors of cyclin-dependent kinases (CDKI) represent possible anticancer drugs. Their anticancer activities have been confirmed in clinical pilot studies. The first synthetic purine inhibitor of cyclin-dependent kinases was olomoucin (Vesely et al., 1994). Since that time a lot of other derivatives were synthesized (Hajduch et al., 1999; Sklenar, 2006). One of the most promising derivatives is the lipophilic roscovitin. In the *Artemia* experimental system we tested the toxicity of some newly synthesized CDKI, and the results compared with the toxicity of olomoucin.

The aim of this study was to test the acute toxicity of roscovitin and three other CDKI, namely TSP 1, TSP 2, and TSP 3 in sea water (salinity 0.9%). As co-solvents were used dimethylsulfoxide (DMSO), polysorbate 80 (TW), or Pluronic F68 (PL). Their toxicities were compared with the control groups (in charts labelled as CG).

The mixture of DMSO and PL occurred inconvenient because of the precipitation of roscovitin that started 24 hrs after dissolving. On the other hand, the mixture of polysorbate 80 and DMSO proved useful and the agents did not precipitate, at all.

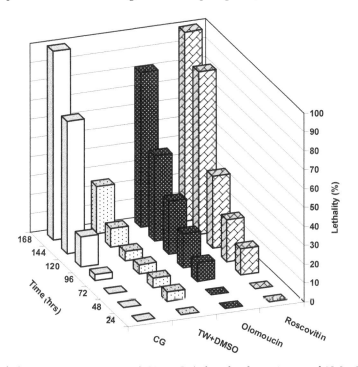

Fig. 3. Effect of olomoucin or roscovitin (100 mg.L^{-1}) dissolved in mixture of 10.0 g.L^{-1} of polysorbate 80 (TW) plus 10.0 g.L^{-1} of dimethylsulfoxide (DMSO) on lethality of *A. franciscana;* CG – control group without any TW or DMSO.

In Fig. 3 we compare the toxicity of olomoucin or roscovitin, both dissolved in mixture of 10.0 g.L^{-1} of polysorbate 80 plus 10.0 g.L^{-1} of DMSO. The final concentration of the tested agents was 100 mg.L^{-1}. The toxicity of these agents was evaluated over 168 hrs. The values of lethality of both agents were significantly different from the toxicity of the control group (TW+DMSO) at the exposures higher than 96 hrs. Both agents, i.e., olomoucin and roscovitin gave the comparable results except for the exposure of 144 hrs, at which the lethality of roscovitin was significantly higher than that of olomoucin.

The simultaneous treatment with DMSO and polysorbate 80 in the concentrations used in our experiments did not cause any deleterious effects on the tested specimens (TW + DMSO). On the contrary, this treatment actually prolonged duration of the test as result of the polysorbate 80 used as energy source by the experimental specimens. Hence, results of the toxicity tests were compared with the control group treated with mixture of DMSO and polysorbate 80 (TW + DMSO).

In the following bar chart (Fig. 4) we compare toxicity of the newly synthesized CDKI, namely TSP 1 (=6-benzylamino-2-(2-aminoethylamino)-9-isopropyl-purine), TSP 2 (=6-benzylamino-2-[(E)-(4-aminocyclohexylamino)]-9-isopropylpurine), and TSP 3 (= 6-benzylamino-2-(3-aminopropylamino)-9-isopropylpurine) with the toxicity of olomoucin. All substances were dissolved in DMSO and used in the concentrations of 100 mg.L^{-1}. While the toxicities of TSP 1 or TSP 3 were comparable with the toxicity of olomoucin, TSP 2 occurred significantly more toxic than olomoucin. The toxicity of TSP 2 was even higher than that of cadmium; hence, this agent was discarded from the further pharmaco-toxicological studies. In general, chromium, cadmium, or zinc are more toxic than olomoucin, roscovitin, TSP 1, or TSP 3 (Sklenar, 2006).

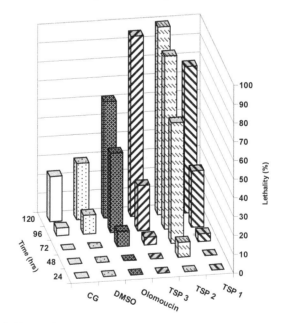

Fig. 4. Comparison of effects of newly synthesised CDKI (TSP 1, TSP 2, and TSP 3) with effects of olomoucin (100 mg.L^{-1}) on lethality of *A. franciscana*. All substances were dissolved in dimethylsulfoxide (DMSO, 15 g.L^{-1}); CG – control group without DMSO.

5.4 Anti-oxidative and pro-oxidative effects of ascorbic acid

The action of ascorbic acid on the oxidative effects of hydrogen peroxide (0.4 g.L⁻¹) was studied. Both, the pro-oxidative and anti-oxidative effects of ascorbic acid were evaluated. The first occurred at the concentration of ascorbic acid 0.3 g.L⁻¹, while the latter at 0.1 g.L⁻¹. The highest anti-oxidative effect was evaluated at the exposure of 96 hrs when the lethality decreased by 34% in comparison with that of hydrogen peroxide per se (Fig. 5).

The search for the antagonists of the oxidative effects of reactive forms of oxygen (free radicals) undoubtedly has been one of the priorities of recent pharmacology. Such antagonistic effects are generally dependant on the concentration of the drug used. In our experiments the ascorbic acid in a concentration of 0.1 g.L⁻¹ partially decreased the oxidative effect of hydrogen peroxide. This finding is in accord with the well-known anti-oxidative efficiency of the ascorbic acid (Young et al., 1992). On the other hand, the higher concentration of ascorbic acid (0.3 g.L⁻¹) operated contrary and increased the final oxidative effect in the simultaneous treatment with 0.4 g.L⁻¹ of hydrogen peroxide. These results are in agreement with the clinical studies showing that the treatments with ascorbic acid at concentrations higher than 1000 mg per day have the pro-oxidative effects, while the effects of the lower concentrations are contrary (Soska et al., 1994). Consequently, the alternative *Artemia* test proved competent for the extensive studies of simultaneous treatments with two agents.

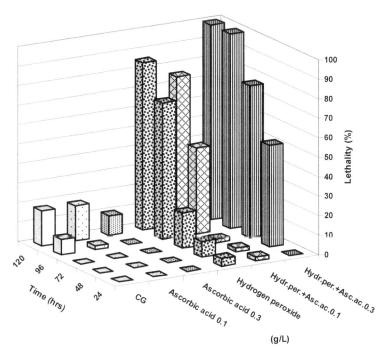

Fig. 5. Effects of simultaneous treatments with ascorbic acid (Asc.ac.; 0.1 or 0.3 g.L⁻¹) and hydrogen peroxide (Hydr.per.; 0.4 g.L⁻¹) on lethality of *A. franciscana*; CG – control group.

5.5 Anti-oxidative effect of *Orobanche flava* plant extract

To the *Orobanche* genus belong annual or perennial parasitic plants that lack chlorophyll, and consequently, fail to perform photosynthesis. They get the nutrients from their host dicotyledonous plants. In our experiments we used *Orobanche flava* (order Scrophulariales, family Orobanchaceae). The pharmacodynamic studies of this plant have shown the positive effects on fatigue, and supporting effects on the immunity system or male potency. From tissues of this plant various chemical substances have been extracted, such as phenylpropanoid glycosides, verbascoside, orobanchoside, tropones, tocochromanoles, fatty acids, phytosterols, carotenoids, or D-mannitol (Erickson, 1969). Some of these agents are supposed to produce anti-oxidative effects. Consequently, effects of the alcoholic extract of this plant on the treatment with hydrogen peroxide were evaluated by the *Artemia* alternative test.

The oxidative effects were induced by hydrogen peroxide in concentrations of 0.4 g.L^{-1} or 0.2 g.L^{-1}. Use of such low concentrations of hydrogen peroxide is on principle in concordance with the real concentrations causing the oxidative effects in vivo. The co-solvent DMSO in concentration of 12.5 g.L^{-1} was used to improve solubility of the plant extract in sea water. In the other experiments, where the effect of the plant extract on the toxicity of DMSO was studied, the latter was used in the concentrations of 50 g.L^{-1} or 100 g.L^{-1}. The alcoholic plant extract was dissolved in DMSO and applied in the concentrations of 0.05, 0.10, 0.25 or 0.50 g.L^{-1}. All concentrations of the plant extract proved non-toxic, or they even decreased the lethality in comparison with the control dishes. At the concentration of 0.5 g.L^{-1} no dead specimens were found. This effect was probably caused by some carbohydrates present in the extract that served as sources of energy for the experimental specimens.

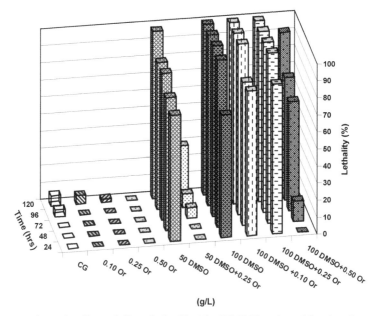

Fig. 6. Decrease in toxic effect of dimethylsulfoxide (DMSO) induced by the plant extract from *Orobanche flava* (Or); CG - control group (no agents); according to Hrbasova (2006).

In the first model experiment we studied the effect of the plant extract on toxicity of the co-solvent per se (Fig. 6). In two experimental combinations (100 g.L^{-1} DMSO + 0.50 g.L^{-1} of plant extract, or 50 g.L^{-1} DMSO + 0.25 g.L^{-1} of plant extract) the toxicity of DMSO was significantly reduced. The other experimental combinations proved rather ineffective.

In the second model experiment the anti-oxidative effects of the plant extract on the oxidative effects of hydrogen peroxide were evaluated. In all simultaneous treatments with the plant extract (0.05 g.L^{-1} or 0.10 g.L^{-1}) plus hydrogen peroxide (0.2 g.L^{-1} or 0.4 g.L^{-1}) the anti-oxidative effects of the plant extract were detected (Fig. 7). While in the combinations with 0.10 g.L^{-1} of the plant extract the anti-oxidative effects were significant, after 96 or 120 hrs, the effect of 0.05 g.L^{-1} occurred positive but insignificant. Thus, we came to the conclusion that the *Artemia* test had proved fully competent for the extensive studies of simultaneous treatments with combinations of drugs.

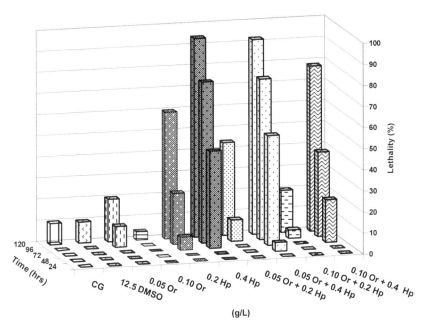

Fig. 7. Decrease in oxidative effect of hydrogen peroxide (Hp; 0.2 g.L^{-1} or 0.4 g.L^{-1}) induced by the plant extract from *Orobanche flava* (Or; 0.05 or 0.10 g.L^{-1}) dissolved in dimethylsulfoxide (DMSO); CG – control group treated with 3% glucose; according to Hrbasova (2006).

5.6 Prolonged treatment with cadmium

Cadmium, as well as zinc or copper, damage SH groups of proteins, resulting in effects analogous to ionizing radiation. These metals bind in tissues to metalothioneins so abundantly, that they may represent up to 11 per cent of the molecular weight of the metalothioneins. If the synthesis of metalothionein is insufficient the toxic effects of cadmium become apparent (Jaywickreme & Chatt, 1990). Lethal treatment of cells, such as lymphocytes, with cadmium may result in the apoptosis (El Azouzi et al., 1994). On the other hand, production of the metalothioneins induced by cadmium may lead to the radioprotective effects (Benova et al., 2006). Genes that control production of the metalothioneins affect also the repair of DNA (Privezencev et al., 1996).

In this test survival of nauplii is prolonged by the treatment with 3% glucose. The aim was to study the effect of cadmium on *Artemia* in the prolonged test system (Fig. 8). The life span of nauplii was prolonged even up to 240 hrs. The mortality of nauplii in the control dishes treated with glucose decreased to only 4% after 216 hrs of exposure. Hence, 3% glucose proved useful for the prolongation of the *Artemia* test up to 10 days. As expected, the toxicity of cadmium increased with increasing concentration and exposure time.

The supplement of glucose to the *Artemia* test system even reduced the toxic effects of cadmium (Dvorak et al., 2005). This finding was significant for the exposure from 24 to 72 hrs and concentrations higher than 50 mg.L^{-1}. The same relationship was valid also for the LC$_{50}$ values expressed in mg.L^{-1} (value without glucose versus value with glucose): at 24 hrs – value 238 versus 482, at 48 hrs – value 250 versus 482, and at 72 hrs – value 195 versus 263. In the same paper we also compared LC$_{50}$ values for three agents used to standardize the microbiotests, namely $K_2Cr_2O_7$, $CdCl_2 . 2H_2O$, and $ZnSO_4 . 7H_2O$. Surprisingly, while the dependence of the toxicity of zinc sulphate on the exposure time was linear, that of the cadmium chloride was logarithmic, and that of potassium dichromate even quadratic.

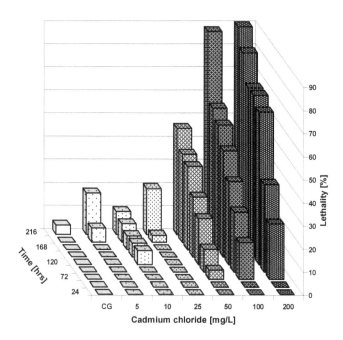

Fig. 8. Effect of cadmium chloride on lethality of *A. franciscana* in test prolonged by glucose (3%), CG - control group supplemented with 3% glucose; according to Dvorak et al. (2005).

6. Conclusion

Eighty years of usage of the *Artemia* species in toxicology testing, and hundreds of papers published all over the world on this theme, have confirmed the exclusivity of this invertebrate genus not only in toxicology or pharmacology, but in biology and medicine as a whole. Our almost twenty years experience with A. *franciscana* have proved that the *Artemia* system is not only convenient for acute toxicity testing, but for extensive dynamic studies, as well, including model experiments with simultaneous treatments with two or more agents of chemical or physical character, as has been demonstrated in this chapter. The *Artemia* tests are fully competent to belong to the group of test systems used for the pre-screening of toxic agents.

7. Acknowledgment

The study was funded by the grant No. MSM6215712402 of the Ministry of Education, Youth and Sports of Czech Republic.

8. References

Abatzopoulos, T.J.; Triantaphyllidis, G.V.; Beardmore, J.A. & Sorgellos, P. (1997). Cyst Membrane Composition as a Discriminant Character in the Genus *Artemia*. (International Study on *Artemia*, LV). *Journal of the Marine Biology Association of the United Kingdom*, Vol.77, No.1, (February 1977), pp. 265-268, ISSN 0025-3154

Amat, F. (1985). *Biologia de Artemia*. Informes Técnicos del Instituto de Investigaciones Pesqueras.

Anderson, D. T. (1967). Larval Development and Segment Formation in the Branchiopod Crustaceans *Limnadia stanley* King (Conchostraca) and *Artemia* salina (L.) (Anostraca). Australian Journal of Zoology, Vol.15, pp. 47-91, ISSN 0004-959X

Bagley, D.M., Waters, D. & Kong, B.M. (1994) Development of a 10-day Chorioallantoic Membrane Vascular Assay as an Alternative to the Draize Rabbit Eye Irritation Test. *Food and Chemical Toxicology*, Vol.32, No.12, (December 1994), pp. 1155–60, ISSN 0278-6915

Balls, M.; Fentem, J. & Jooint, E. (1992). Issues: Animal Experiments. Hobson Publishing, Cambridge, pp. 2-15

Barahona, M.V. & Sánchez-Fortún, S. (1998). Toxicity of Carbamates to the Brine Shrimp *Artemia salina* and the Effect of Atropine, Iso-ompa and 2-PAM on Carbaryl Toxicity. *Environmental Pollution*, Vol.104, No.3, (1999), pp. 469-476, ISSN 0269-7491

Barahona-Gomariz, M.V.; Sanz-Barrera, F.; Sánchez-Fortún, S. (1994). Acute Toxicity of Organic Solvents on *Artemia salina*. *Bulletin of Environmental Contamination and Toxicology*, Vol.52, No.2, (May 1994), pp. 766-771, ISSN 0007-4861

Beattie, K.A.; Ressler, J.; Wiegand, C., Krause, E., Codd, G.A.; Steinberg, C.E.W. & Pflugmacher, S. (2003). Comparative Effects and Metabolism of Two Microcystins and Nodularin in the Brine Shrimp *Artemia salina*. *Aquatic Toxicology*, Vol.62, (February 2003), No.3, pp. 219-226, ISSN 0166-445X

Benova, K.; Dvorak, P.; Falis, M. & Danova, D. (2006). Elimination of Negative Effects of cadmium in *Artemia franciscana* by Exposure to Ionizing Radiation. *Folia Veterinaria,* Vol.50, No.3, (Supplementum 2006), pp. 21-22, ISSN 03010724

Benesch, R. (1969). Zur Ontogenie und Morphologie von *Artemia salina* L. *Zoologische Jahrbucher, Abteilung für Anatomie and Ontogenie der Tiere,* Vol.86, pp. 307-458

Blaise, C. (1991) Microbiotests in Aquatic Toxicology: Characteristics, Utility and Prospects. *Environmental Toxicology and Water Quality,* Vol.6, No.2, (May 1991), pp. 145–155, ISSN 1053-4725

Boone, E. & Baas-Becking, L.G.M. (1931). Salt Effects on Eggs and Nauplii of *Artemia salina* L. The Journal of General Physiology. July 20, pp. 753-763. Available from http://jpg.rupress.org/content/14/6/753.full.pdf

Boroughs, H.; Townsley, S.J. & Ego, W. (1958) The Accumulation of Y^{90} from an Equilibrium Micture of $Sr^{90} - Y^{90}$ by *Artemia salina.* (L), Vol.3, No.4, pp. 413-317. Available from http://www.aslo.org/lo.org/lo/toc/vol_3/issue_4/0413.pdf

Brix, K.V.; Cardwell, R.D.; Adams, W.J. (2003). Chronic Toxicity of Arsenic to the Great Salt Lake Brine Shrimp, *Artemia franciscana. Ecotoxicology and Environmental Safety.* Vol. 54, No.2, (February 2003), pp. 169-175, ISSN 0147-6513

Brix, K.V.; Gerdes, R.M.; Adams, W.J. & Grosell, J. (2006). Effects of Copper, Cadmium, and Zinc on the hatching success of brine shrimp (*Artemia franciscana*). *Archives of Environmental Contamination and Toxicology.* Vol.51, No.4, (November 2006), pp. 580-583, ISSN 0090-4341

Browne, T. A. (1980). Acute Response versus Reproductive Performance in five Strains of Brine Shrimp exposed to Copper Sulphate. *Marine Environmental Research.* Vol.3, pp. 185-193, ISSN 0141-1136

Browne, R. A. (1992). Population Genetics and Ecology of *Artemia*: Insights into Parthenogenetic Reproduction. *Trends in Ecology and Evolution,* Vol.7, No.7, pp. 232-237, ISSN 0169-5347

Browne, R.A.; Li, M.; Wanigasekera, G.; Simonek, S.; Brownlee, D.; Eiband, G. & Cowan, J. (1991). Ecological, Physiological and Genetic Divergence of Sexual and Asexual (diploid and polyploid) Brine Shrimp (*Artemia*). In: Menon, J. (ed.): *Advances in Ecology.* Vol. 1. Trivandrum, India: Council of Research Integration. pp. 41-52

Cáceres, A.; López, B.; González, S.; Berger, I.; Tada, I. & Maki, J. (1998). Plants used in Guatemala for the Treatment of Protozoal Infections. I. Screening of Activity to Bacteria, Fungi, and American Trypanosomes of 13 Native Plants. *Journal of Ethnopharmacology,* Vol.62, No.3, (October 1998), pp. 195-202, ISSN 0378-8741

Calleja, M.C. & Persoone, G. (1992). Cyst-based Toxicity Tests: 4. The Potential of Ecotoxicological Tests for the Prediction of Acute Toxicity in Man as Evaluated on the First ten Chemicals of the MEIC Programme. *Alternatives to Laboratory Animals,* Vol.20, No.3, p. 396-405, ISSN 02611929

Dattilo, A.M.; Bracchini, L.; Carlini, L.; Loiselle, S. & Rossi. C. (2005). Estimate of the Effects of Ultraviolet Radiation on the Mortality of *Artemia franciscana* in Naupliar and Adult Stages. *International Journal of Biometeorology,* Vol.49, No.6, (July 2005), pp. 388-395, ISSN 0020-7128

Dvorak, P. (1995). Modified *A. salina* Test for Evaluation of Interactions of Heterogenous agents (In Czech). In: *Toxicita a biodegradabilita odpadu a latek vyznamnych ve vodnim prostredi. Sbornik refereatu ze 7. konference, Milenovice.* Vyzkumny ustav rybarsky a hydrobiologicky, Vodnany, pp. 25-29. ISBN 80-85887-02-9

Dvorak, P.; Benova, K. (2002). The Investigation of Interactions of Low Doses of Ionizing Radiation and Risk Factors by Means of *Artemia salina* Biotest. *Folia Veterinaria*, Vol. 46, No. 4, pp. 195-197, ISSN 03010724

Dvorak, P.; Sucman, E. & Benova, K. (2005). The Development of a Ten-day Bio-test using *Artemia salina* Nauplii. *Biologia*, Vol.60, No.5, (September 2005), pp. 593-597, ISSN 0006-3088

Easter, S.S. & Hutchinson, F. (1961). Effects of Radiations of Different LET on *Artemia* Eggs. *Radiation Research*, Vol.15, No.3, pp. 333-340, ISSN 0033-7587

El Azzouzi, B.; Tsangaris, G.R.; Pollegrini, O.; Manuel, Y.; Benveniste, J. & Thomas, Y. (1994). Cadmium Induces Apoptosis in a Human T Cell Line. *Toxicology*, Vol.88, No.1-3, (March 1994), pp. 127-139, ISSN 0300-483X

Erickson, R. L. (1969). Hot Watter–Soluble Glycosides: Location in the Tissue of *Populus grandidentata* Bark. (Doctor's Dissertation). The Institute of Paper Chemistry, Appleton, Wisconsin. June 1969. pp. 66

Fentem, J. & Balls, M. (1993). Biology now! In: *Developing Alternatives to Animal Experimentation.* Hobson Publishing, Cambridge

Fouradzieva, S.; Dittrat, F.; Lukavsky, J. (1995). Toxicity of Trichlorethylen on Green Algae (In Czech). In: *Toxicita a biodegradabilita odpadu a latek vyznamnych ve vodnim prostredi. Sbornik refereatu ze 7. konference, Milenovice.* Vyzkumny ustav rybarsky a hydrobiologicky, Vodnany, pp. 38-41, ISBN 80-85887-02-9

George-Ares, A.; Febbo,E.J.; Letinski, D.J.; Yarusinsky, J.; Safadi, R.S. & Aita, A.F. (2003) Use of Brine Shrimp (*Artemia*) in Dispersant Toxicity Tests: Some Caveats. In: *Proceedings of International Oil Spill Conference*, 2003

Gilchrist, B.M. (1960). Growth and Form of the Brine Shrimp *Artemia salina*. *Proceedings of the Zoological Society of London*, Vol.152, No.946, pp. 221-235, ISSN 0962-8452

Granade, H.R.; Cheng, P.C. & Doorenbos, N.J. (1976). Ciguatera, I. Brine Shrimp (*Artemia salina* L.) Larval Assay for Ciguatera toxins. *Journal of Pharmaceutical Sciences*, Vol. 65, No.9, pp. 1414-1415, ISSN 0022-3549

Graul, E.H.; Ruther, W.; Heinrich, W.; Allkofer, O.C.; Kaiser, R.; Pfohl, R.; Schopper, E.; Henig, G.; Schott, J.U. & Bucker, H. (1975). Radiobiological Results of the Biostack Experiment on Board Apollo 16 and 17. *Life Sciences Research in Space*, Vol.13, pp. 153–159, ISSN 0006-3185

Grosch, D.S. & Erdman, H.E. (1955). X-ray Effects on Adult *Artemia*. *Biological Bulletin*, Vol. 108, No.3, pp. 277 282. ISSN: 0006 3185

Guerra, R. (2001). Ecotoxicological and Chemical Evaluation of Phenolic Compounds in Industrial Effluents. *Chemosphere*, Vol.44, No.8, (September 2001), pp. 1737-1747, ISSN 0045-6535

Hadjispyrou, S.; Kungolos, A. & Anagnostopoulos, A. (2001). Toxicity, Bioaccumulation, and Interactive Effects of Organotin, Cadmium and Chromium on *Artemia franciscana. Ecotoxicology and Environmental Safety.* Vol.49, No.2, (June 2001), pp. 179-186, ISSN 0147-6513

Hajduch, M.; Havlicek, L.; Vesely, J.; Novotný, R.; Mihal, V. & Strnad M. (1999). Synthetic Cyclin-dependent Kinase Inhibitors - New Generation of Potent Anti-cancer Drugs.

Conference Information: 3rd International Symposium on Drug Resistance in Leukemia and Lymphoma, (March 1998), Amsterdam, Netherlands Source: Drug resistance in leukemia and lymphoma III, Book Series: *Advances in Experimental Medicine and Biology*, Vol.457, pp. 341-353, ISSN 0065-2598, ISBN 0-306-46055-6

Hayes, W.J. (1991). Dosage and other Factors Influencing Toxicity. In: *Handbook of Pesticide Toxicology. General Principles*. Hayes, W.J.Jr., Laws, E.R. (Ed.), Academic Press. Vol. 1, pp. 39-97, ISBN 0-12-334161-2

Heinrich, W. (1977). Calculation of the Radiobiological Effects of Heavy Ions on Eggs of *Artemia salina* flown in the Biostack Experiments. *Life Sciences Research in Space*, Vol. 15, pp. 157–163, ISSN 0006-3185

Hentschel, E. (1968). Die postembryonalen Entwicklungsstadien von *Artemia salina* bei verschiedene temperaturen (Anostraca, Crustaceae). *Zoologischer Anzeiger*, Vol.180, pp. 73-384, ISSN 00445231

Hertel, H. (1980). The Compound Eye of *Artemia salina* (Crustacea). I. Fine Structure when Light and Dark Adapted. *Zoologische Jahrbucher für allgemeine Zoologie und Physiologie der Tiere*, Vol. 84, No.1, pp.1-14, ISSN 0044-5185

Hlywka, J.J.; Beck, M.M. & Bullerman, L.B. (1997). The Use of the Chicken Embryo Screening Test and Brine Shrimp (*Artemia salina*) Bioassays to Assess the Toxicity of Fumonisin B_1 Mycotoxin. *Food and Chemical Toxicology*, Vol. 35, No.10-11, (Ocrober-November 1997), pp. 991-999, ISSN 0278-6915

Horowitz, M. (1970). Notes on Bioassay Techniques for Several Soil-applied Substituted Ureas. *Israel Journal of agricultural Research*, Vol.21, No.2, pp. 281-284, IDS Number G2245

Hrbasova, L. (2006). Evaluation of Anti-oxidative Effects of Plant Extract of *Orobanche flava* by *Artemia salina* Biotest (In Czech). *Graduation thesis*. University of Veterinary and Pharmaceutical Science, Faculty of Pharmacy, Brno, p. 41

Huska, D.; Krizkova, S.; Beklova, M.; Havel, L.; Zahnalek, J.; Diopan, V.; Adam, V.; Zeman, L.; Babula, P. & Kizek, R. (2008). Influence of Cadmium(II) Ions and Brewery Sludge on Metallothinein Level in Earthworms (*Eisenia fetida*) – Biotransforming of Toxic Wastes. *Sensors*, Vol.8, No.2, (February 2008), pp. 1039-1047, ISSN 1424-8220

Kikuchi, S. (1971). The Fine Structure of the Alimentary Canal of the Brine Shrimp, *Artemia salina*: The Midgut. *Annual Report of Iwate Medical University, School of Liberal Arts and Sciences*, Vol.7, p. 15-47

Kinghorn, A. D.; Haarjes, K.K. & Doorenbos, N.J. (1977). Screening Procedure for Phorbol Esters using Brine Shrimp (*Artemia salina*) Larvae. *Journal of Pharmaceutical Sciences*, Vol.66, No.9, pp. 1362-1363, ISSN 0022-3549

Knulst, J. & Sodergren, A. (1994). Occurence and Toxicity of Persistent Pollutants in Surface Microlayers Near an Incineration Plant. *Chemosphere*, Vol.29, No.6, (September 1994), pp. 1339-1347, ISSN 0045-6535

Kratky, B.A. & Warren, G.F. (1971). The use of three simple rapid Bioassays on forty-two Herbicides. *Weed Research*, Vol.11, No.4, pp. 257-262, ISSN 0043-1737

Jacob, S.W. & Herschler, R. (1986). Pharmacology of DMSO. *Cryobiolgy*, Vol.23, No.1, (February 1986), pp.14-27, ISSN 0011-2240

Jayawickreme, C.K. & Chatt, A. (1990). Studies on Zinc and Cadmium – bound Proteins in Bovine Kidneys by Biochemical and Neutron Activation Techniques. *Biological Trace Element Research*, Vol.26-27, (July-December 1990), pp. 503-512, ISSN 0163-4984

Martin, J.W. & Davis, G.E. (2001). An Updated Classification of the Recent Crustacea. In: *Natural History Museum of Los Angeles County, Science Series 39*, Brown, K.V. (Ed.) (December 2001), pp. 1-124 , ISSN 1-891276-27-1

Mayorga, P.; Pérez, K.R.; Cruz, S.M. & Cáceres, S. (2010). Comparison of Bioassays using the Anostracan Crustaceans *Artemia salina* and *Thamnocephalus platyurus* for Plant Extract Toxicity Screening. *Revista Brasileira de Farmacognosia-Brazilian Journal of Pharmacognosy*, Vol.20, No.6, (December 2010), pp. 897-903, ISSN 0102-695X

Michael, A.S.; Thompson, C.B. & Abramovitz, M. (1956). *Artemia salina* as a Test Organism for Bioassay. *Science*, Vol.123, No.3194, pp. 464, ISSN 0036-8075

Nalecz-Jawecki, G.; Grabinska-Sota, E.; & Narkiewicz, P. (2003). The Toxicity of Cationic Surfactants in four Bioassays. *Ecotoxicology and Environmental Safety*, Vol. 54, No.1, (January 2003), pp. 87-91, ISSN 0147-6513

Nunes, B. S.; Carvalho, F. D. ; Guilhermino, L. M. & Van Stappen, G. (2006). Use of the Genus *Artemia* in Ecotoxicity Testing. *Environmental Pollution*, Vol.144, No.2, (November 2006), pp. 453-462, ISSN 0269-7491

Okamura, H., Aoyama, I., Liu, D., Maguire, R.J., Pacepavicius, G.J. & Lau, Y.L. (2000). Fate and Ecotoxicity of the New Antifouling Compound Irgarol 1051 in the Aguatic Environment. *Water Research*, Vol. 34, No.14, (October 2000), pp. 3523-3530, ISSN 0043-1354

Oliveira-Filha, E.C. & Paumgartten, F.J.R. (2000). Toxiticity of *Euphorbia milii* Latex and Niclosamide to Snails and Nontarget Aquatic Species. *Ecotoxicology and Environmental Safety*, Vol.46, No.3, (July 2000), pp. 342-350, ISSN 0147-6513

Panigrahi, S. (1993. Bioassay of mycotoxins using terrestrial and aquatic, animal and plant species. *Food Chemistry and Toxicology*, Vol.31, No.10, (OCT 1993), pp. 767-790, ISSN 0278-6915

Parra, L.A.; Silva, Y.; Guerra, S.I.; Iglesias, B.L. (2001). Comparative Study of the Assay of *Artemia salina* L. and the Estimate of the Medium Lethal Dose (LD$_{50}$) Value in Mice, to Determine Oral Acute Toxicity of Plant Extracts. *Phytomedicine*, Vol.8, No.5, pp. 395-400, ISSN 09447113

Pazourek, J. (1992). Simulation of biological systems (In Czech). Grada, ISBN 80-85623-13-7, Praha, Czech Republic, pp. 284

Persoone, G., Wells, P.G. (1987). *Artemia* in Aquatic Toxicology: A Review. In: *Artemia Research and its Applications. Morphology, Genetics, Strain Characterization, Toxicology.* Sorgellos P.; Bengtson, D.A.; Decleir, W. and Jaspers, E. (Eds.).Vol. I. Universa Press, Wetteren, Belgium

Petrucci, F.; Caimi, S.; Mura, G. & Caroli, S. (1995). *Artemia* as a Test Organism of Environmental Contamination by Trace Elements. *Microchemical Journal*, Vol.51, No.1-2, (February-April 1995), pp. 181-186, ISSN 0026-265X

Pilla, E. J. S. & Beardmore, J. A. (1994). Genetic and Morphometric Differentiation in Old World Bisexual Species of *Artemia* (the brine shrimp). *Heredity*, Vol..73, No.1, (July 1994), pp. 47-56, ISSN 0018-067X

Privezencev, K.V.; Sirota, N.P.; & Gaziev, A.I. (1996). Effect of Simultaneous Treatment of Cadmium and Gamma-radiation on Damage and Repair of DNA in Lymphoide Tissues of Mice (In Russian). *Radiacionnaja biologija, radioekologija*. Vol.36, No.2, pp. 234-239, ISSN 0869-8031

Richter, J.A. & Goldstein, A. (1970). The Effects of Morphine-like Compounds on the Light Responses of the Brine Shrimp *Artemia salina*. *Psychopharmacologia*, Vol.17, No.4, pp. 327-337, IDS Number G7382

Robinson, A.B.; Manly, K.F.; Anthony, M.P.; Catchpool, J.F. & Pauling, L. (1965). Anesthesia of *Artemia* Larvae: Method for Quantitative Study. *Science*, Vol.149, No.3689, pp. 1255-1258, ISSN 0036-8075

Rowe, R.C., Sheskey, P.J. & Owen, S.C. (2006). Handbook of Pharmaceutical Excipients. 5. Royal Pharmaceutical Society of Great Britain, 918 p., ISBN 0-85369-618-7, London, Great Britain

Ruppert, E.E. & Barnes, R.D. (1994). *Invertebrate Zoology 6*, Saunders College Publishing, ISBN 0-03-026668-8, New York , USA

Ruther, W.; Graul, E.H.; Heinrich, W.; Allkofer, O.C.; Kaiser, R. & Cuer, P. (1974). Preliminary Results on the Action of Cosmic Heavy Ions on the Development of Eggs of *Artemia salina*. *Life Sciences Research in Space*, Vol.12, pp. 69–74, ISSN 0006-3185

Sarabia, R.; Varó, I.; Torreblanca, A.; Del Ramo, J.J.; Pastor, A.; Amat, F. & Díaz-Mayans, J. (1998a). Accumulation of Cadmium in several Crains of *Artemia*. *Cuadernos de Investigación Biológica*. Vol.20, pp.435-438

Sarabia, R.; Torreblanca, A.; Del Ramo, J.J. & Díaz-Mayans, J. (1998b). Effects of low Mercury Concentration Exposure on Hatching, Growth and Survival in the *Artemia* Strain La Mata Parthenogenetic Diploid. *Comparative Biochemistry and Physiology A-Molecular & integrative Physiology*. Vol.120, No.1, (May 1998), pp. 93-97, ISSN 1095-6433

Sarabia, R.; Del Ramo, J.; Varó, I.; Díaz-Mayans & Torreblanca A. (2002). Comparing the Acute Exposure to Cadmium Toxicity of Nauplii from Different Populations of *Artemia*. *Environmental Toxicology and Chemistry*. Vol.21, No.2, (February 2002), pp. 437-444, ISSN 0730-7268

Sarabia, R.; Varó, I.; Amat, F. Pastor, A.; Del Ramo, J.J.; Díaz-Mayans, J. & Torreblanca, A. (2006). Comparative Toxicokinetics of Cadmium in *Artemia*. *Archives of Environmental Contamination and Toxicology*, Vol.50, No.1, (January 2006), pp. 111-120, ISSN 0090-4341

Schmidt, R. (1985). Optical Motility Test for the Detection of Trichothecenes using Brine Shrimps. *Mycotoxin Research*, Vol. 1, pp. 25-29

Sklenar, Z. (2006). Evaluation of Toxicity and Morphological Changes Induced by Purine Inhibitors of Cyclin-dependent Kinases (In Czech). Dissertation thesis. Faculty of Veterinary Hygiene and Ecology. University of Veterinary and Pharmaceutical Sciences, Brno. 138 p.

Soares, A.M.V.M.; Baird, D.J. & Calow, P. (1992). Interclonal Variation in the Performace of *Daphnia magna* Straus in Chronic Bioassays. *Environmental Toxicology and Chemistry*, Vol.11, No.10, (October 1992), pp. 1477-1483, ISSN 0730-7268

Solis, P.N.; Wright, C.W.; Anderson, M.M.; Gupta, M.P. & Phillipson, J.D. (1993). A Microwell Cytotoxicity Assay using *Artemia salina* (Brine Shrimp). *Planta Medica*, Vol. 59, No.3, (June 1993), pp. 250-252, ISSN 0032-0943

Song, M.Y. & Brown, J.J. (1998). Osmotic Effects as a Factor Modifying Insecticide Toxicity on *Aedes* and *Artemia*. *Ecotoxicology and Environmental Safety*, Vol.41, No.2, (October 1998), pp. 195-202, ISSN 0147-6513

Sorgeloos, P.; Remiche-van der Wielen, C. & Persoone G. (1978). The Use of *Artemia* Nauplii for Toxicity Tests A Critical Analysis. *Ecotoxicology and Environmental Safety*, Vol.2, pp. 249-255, ISSN 0147-6513

Soska, V.; Zechmeister, A.; Lojek, A. & Podrouzkova, B. (1994). Effect of L-ascorbic acid on Lipids and Free Radicals in Blood of Patients with Hyperlipoproteinemia (In Czech). *Klinicka Biochemie a Metabolismus*, Vol.23, No.2, pp. 86-88, ISSN 1210-7921

Tong, Z.; Hongjun, J. & Huailan, Z. (1996). Quality Criteria of Acrylonitrile for the Protection of Aquatic Life in China. *Chemosphere*, Vol.32, pp. 2083-2093, ISSN 0045-6535

Touraki, M., Nikopas, I. & Kastritsis, C. (1999). Bioaccumulation of Trimethoprim, Sulfamethoxazole and N-acetyl-sulfamethoxazole in *Artemia nauplii* and Residual Kinetics in Seabass Larvae after Repeated Oral Dosing of Medicated Nauplii. *Aquaculture*, Vol.175, No.1-2, (April 1999), pp. 15-30, ISSN 0044-8486

Triantaphyllidis, G.V.; Pilla, E.J.S.; Thomas, K.M.; Abatzopoulos, T.J.; Beardmore, J.A. & Sorgeloos. P. (1994). International Study on *Artemia*. 52. Incubation of Artemia Cyst Samples at High Temperatures Reveals Mixed Nature with *Artemia franciscana* Cysts. *Journal of Experimental Marine Biology and Ecology*, Vol.183, No.2, (November 1994), pp. 273-282, ISSN 0022-0981

Vanhaecke, P.; & Persoone, G. (1981). Report on an Intercalibration Exercise on a Short-term Standard Toxicity Test with *Artemia* Nauplii (ARC-test). *Institut Snational de la Santé et de la Recherche Médicale (INSERM)*, Vol.106. pp. 359-376

Vanhaecke, P.; Persoone, G.; Claus, C. & Sorgeloos, P. (1980). Research on the Development of a Short-term Standard Toxicity Test with *Artemia*. The Brine Shrimp *Artemia*. In: *Exology, Culturing. Use in Aquaculture*. Vol.1, pp. 263-285

Van Wezel, A.P.; Van Vlaardingen, P.; Posthumus, R.; Crommentuijn, G.H.; Sijm, D.T.H.M. (2000). Environmental Risk Limits for Two Phthalates, with Special Emphasis on Endocrine Disruptive Properties. *Ecotoxicology and Environmental Safety*, Vol.46, No.3, (July 2000), pp. 305-321, ISSN 0147-6513

Varó, I.; Navarro, J.C.; Amat, F. & Guilhermino, L. (2002). Characterisation of Cholinesterases and Evaluation of the Inhibitory Potential of Chlorpyrifos and Dichlorvos to *Artemia salina* and *Artemia parthenogenetica*. *Chemosphere*, Vol.18, No.6, (August 2002), pp. 563-569, ISSN 0045-6535

Varó, I.; Taylor, A.C.; Ferrando, M.D. & Amat, F. (1997). Effect of Endosulfan Pesticide on the Oxygen Consumption Rates of Nauplii of Different Spanish Strains of *Artemia*. *Journal of Environment Science and Health-Part B.: Pesticides, Food Contaminants and Agricultural Wastes*, Vol.32, No.3, pp. 363-375, ISSN 0360-1234

Vesely, J.; Havlicek, L.; Strnad, M.; Blow, J.J.; Donella-Deana, A.; Pinna, L.; Letham, D.S., Kato, J.; Detivaud, L.; Leclerc, S. & Meijer, L. (1994). Inhibition of Cyclin-dependent Kinases by Purine Analogues. *European Journa of Biochememistry*, Vol.224, No.2, (September 1994), pp. 771-786, ISSN 0014-2956

Vezie, C.; Sivonen, K.; Brient, L.; Bertru, G. & Lefeuvre, J.C. (1996). Development of Toxic Cyanobacteria in Western France-Detection of Toxicity with *Artemia salina* Tests. *Annales de Limnologie-International Journal of Limnology*, Vol.32, No.2, pp. 123-128, ISSN 0003-4088

Young, I.S.; Torney, J.J. & Trimble, E.R. (1992). The Effect of Ascorbate Supplementation on Oxidative Stress in the Streptozotocin Diabetic Rat. *Free Radical Biology and Medicine*, Vol.13, No.1, (July 1992), pp. 41-46, ISSN 0891-5849

Zillioux, E.J; Foulk, H. R.; Prager, J.C. & Cardin, J.A. (1973). Using *Artemia* to Assay Oil Dispersant Toxicities. *Journal Water Pollution Control Federation*, Vol. 45, No.11, pp. 2389-2396, ISSN 0043-1303

6

Comparative Genotoxicity Analysis of Heavy Metal Contamination in Higher Plants

Sumer Aras, Semra Soydam Aydin,
Didem Aksoy Körpe* and Çiğdem Dönmez
Ankara University
Turkey

1. Introduction

Heavy metal pollution basically results from natural sources like volcanic eruptions, weathering of rocks and anthropogenic sources like mining. These activities are significantly increased in the past few decades as a result of burning of fossil fuels, industrial activities, automotive emissions, use of metal-enriched materials, mining, farm manures, wastewater irrigation, sewage sludge, pesticide usage, industrial and domestic wastes and many other factors. Heavy metals may enter the food chain as a result of their uptake by edible plants, thus, the determination of heavy metals in environmental samples is very important. For screening and monitoring the impacts of heavy metals, higher plants which provide useful genetic system, have been used as a biomonitor/bioindicator of cytogenetic and mutagenic effects (Constantin & Owens, 1982; Grant, 1994, Kachenko et al. 2004; Alirzaveya et al. 2006).

Plants are used as biomonitor / bioindicator of pollution and the major advantages of them are the following; they are eukaryotes and like animals, are able to process complex pollutant molecules (promutagen - mutagen), there is a positive correlation with mammalian cytogenetic assays for mutagenesis, easy to grow, resistant to environmental stresses, do not contaminate easily, allow assays of a range of environmental conditions, also with cultured cells; used for outdoor monitoring (Sandermann, 1994). Hence, the usage of plants as bioindicator in ecotoxicology have been reported in several studies (Grant, 1994; Knasmuller et al., 1998).

2. Effects of heavy metal on plants and defense mechanism

Some metals e.g. Mn, Cu, Zn, Mo and Ni are essential for normal growth and development of plants at appropriate concentrations as cofactors and or required for structural and catalytic components of proteins and enzymes (Moustakas et al., 1994; Nedelkoska & Doran, 2000). However, toxic levels of heavy metal ions induce several cellular stress responses and damages different cellular components such as membranes, proteins and DNA (Patra et al., 1998; Waisberg et al., 2003; Jimi et al., 2004). When heavy metals accumulate in plant tissues, they alterate in various vital growth processes, such as mineral nutrition (Greger & Lindberg, 1987, Ouzounidou et al., 1992) transpiration (Poschenrieder et. al., 1989), photosynthesis (Lidon & Henriques, 1991, enzyme activities-related to metabolism

---

* Current addess: Başkent University, Turkey

(Nussbaum et. al., 1988) and biosynthesis of chlorophyll (Lidon & Henriques,1991), nucleic acids (Shah & Dubey, 1995; Doncheva et. al., 1996) and seed germination (Ouzounidou et. al., 1992).

Lead (Pb) naturally occurs in uncontaminated soils are generally in the range of 20 to 50 mg kg⁻¹ (Nriagu, 1978). In industrialized areas, Pb up to 1000 mg kg⁻¹ or above has been recorded (Angelone & Bini, 1992). Although it is not an essential element for plants, it gets easily absorbed and accumulates in different parts of plants, causes anatomical changes by binding with essential enzymes and cellular components and inactivates them in primary leaves and decreases the number of epidermal cells/mm and growth parameters (Chaudhry & Qurat-ul-Ain, 2003). Toxicity of Pb in plants causes a number of toxicity symptoms as stunted growth, chlorosis, and blackening of root system and inhibits photosynthesis, upsets mineral nutrition and water balance, changes hormonal status and affects membrane structure and permeability (Sharma a& Dubey, 2005).

Copper (Cu) known to be an essential micronutrient for plant nutrition is generally occurs in the range of 20-30 ppm in uncontaminated areas and sediments and less than 2 ppb in natural waters (Nriagu, 1979; Salomons & Forstner, 1984; Moore & Ramamoorthy, 1984; Baccini, 1985). Cu ions play a significant role in cell metabolism and also catalyse the redox reactions in which 0_2 is the electron acceptor, being reduced to H_2O_2 or H_2O (Gupta, 1979). However its deleterious effects usually arise toxic levels in mining areas (higher than 2000 ppm) (Freedman & Hutchinson, 1980; Humphreys & Nicholls, 1984). Excesses of Cu ions in plant tissues may induce a wide range of biochemical effects and metabolic disturbances which are responsible for a strong inhibition of growth, sometimes accompanied by anomalous development (Sommer, 1931; Lipman & McKinney 1931) and block photosynthetic electron transport at the reducing site of photosystem I and at the oxidizing site of photosystem II (Arnon & Stout 1939).

In natural soils cadmium (Cd) content is estimated to be about 0.06-0.50 mg/kg. Also, accession of Cd to environment and its several potentially toxic consequences in soil–plant–animal–human system have increased due to industrial, agricultural and municipal activities (Baker et al., 1979; Qadir et al., 2000). Cd is easily translocated from plant roots to stems and leaves (Yang et al., 1998), and interfere with physiological processes, resulting in declined productivity (Florijn & Van Beusichem, 1993) and harness photosynthetic activity, chlorophyll content, plant growth and induce oxidative stress (Zhou & Huang, 2001; Yi and Ching, 2003; Zhou et al., 2003). Cd stress leads to protein degradation through amino acid metabolism resulting in decreased plant growth (Rai & Raizada, 1988) and inhibits the activity of enzymes such as nitrate reductase and nitrite reductase is reported by Boussama et al. (1999a, 1999b). Previous reports indicated that Cd can cause significant reduction in the germination rate in *Triticum* and *Cucumis* (Munzuroglu & Geckil, 2002) or inhibit germination and the growth of *Arabidopsis* embryos (Li et al., 2005).

Zinc (Zn) is essential microelement that is indispensable for normal plant growth. The essentiality of Zn in low concentration for root and stem elongation was shown in previous researches (Mazé, 1915; Sommer & Lipman, 1926; Skoog, 1940). But at high concentrations, it is toxic for plants like cadmium, lead and copper. Zn toxicity occurs in plants by contaminated soils with mining and smelting activities (Chaney, 1993). Also genetic variations in sensitivity to Zn toxicity has been mapped in plants (Dong et al., 2006).

Plants could develop efficient and specific physio-biochemical mechanisms and overcome environmental stress (Sandalio et al., 2001). For instance, some of them store toxic metals in roots in order to prevent the dispersal of ions into the other parts of the plant (Fernandes & Henriques, 1991). Plants tolerate metallic stress by developing the following defence mechanisms.

- Excretion of complex compounds that reduce metal availability in the soil or in the water.
- Metal exclusion through selective uptake of elements
- Metal retention in the roots, preventing its translocation to the shoot.
- Metal immobilization in the cell wall.
- Metal accumulation in vacuoles and inclusions.
- Increased production of intracellular metal-binding compounds.
- Development of metal-tolerant enzymes

Heavy metal toxicity effects biological molecules, for example, when metals binds to S group, blocks the active site of enzyme, and may cause conformational changes in enzymes, disrupts the cellular homeostasis and cause oxidative damage by generating reactive oxygen species (ROS) such as singlet oxygen, hydrogen peroxide, hydroxyl radical which cause lipid peroxidation, membrane defects and unstability of enzymes in higher plants (Webber, 1981; Freedman & Hutchinson, 1981; Aust et al., 1985). Chloroplast, mitochondrial and plasma membrane are linked to electron transport and generate ROS as by products (Becana et al., 2000). Their presence causes oxidative damage to the biomolecules such as lipids, proteins and nucleic acids (Kanazawa et al., 2000). A variety of abiotic stresses including drought, salinity, extreme temperatures, high irradiance, UV light, nutrient deficiency, air pollutants, metallic stress etc. lead to formation of ROS and result directly or indirectly in molecular damage (Lin & Kao, 1999). The regulation of ROS is a crucial process to avoid unwanted cellular cytotoxicity and oxidative damage (Halliwell & Gutteridge, 1989). Effects and results of ROS (Reactive Oxygen Species) are shown in Figure 1.

To scavenge ROS and avoid oxidative damage plants posses the antioxidative enzymes superoxide dismutase, peroxidase and catalase (Kanazawa et al., 2000). SOD plays a determinant role in protection against the toxic effects of oxidative stress by scavenging superoxide radicals and providing their conversion into oxygen and hydrogen peroxide (McCord & Fridovich, 1969). Four different classes of SOD have been distinguished depending on the metal at the active center, manganese (Mn), iron (Fe), copper (Cu) and zinc (Zn) (Miller & Sorkin, 1997). Previous studies with plants have demonstrated that, most of the SODs are intracellular enzymes. A class of SODs consist with Cu (II) and Zn (II) at active site (Cu/Zn SOD), another Mn(III) at active site (MnSOD), and with Fe (III) or Ni (III) at the active site (FeSOD). Cu/Zn SODs are generally found in the cytosol of eukaryotic cells and chloroplasts; membrane associated MnSODs are found in mitochondria and also reported in chloroplasts and peroxisomes in some plants; the dimeric FeSODs which is lacking in animals have been reported in chloroplasts of some but not all, plants (Salin & Bridges 1980; Del Rio et al. 1983; Droillard & Paulin 1990; Van Camp 1994; Fridovich, 1995).

Peroxidases are heme-containing monomeric glycoproteins that utilize either H_2O_2 or O_2 to oxidaze a wide variety of molecules (Yoshida, 2002). They are located in cytosol, vacuole, cell wall as well as in extra cellular space and use guaiacol as electron donor, utilise H_2O_2 in the oxidation of various inorganic and organic substrates (Asada et al., 2006).

Catalase is in age dependent manner and scavenge H_2O_2 generated during the photorespiration and β-oxidation of fatty acids (Lin & Kao, 2000) and one of the crucial antioxidant enzyme that scavenge ROS generated under stress conditions in plants. It catalyzes the conversion of H_2O_2 to O_2 and H_2O, in this way prevents longer H_2O_2 action which may lead to cell disturbances and DNA damages. The antioxidative responses of catalase to heavy metal stress found predominantly in peroxisomes. Hence, researchers have been investigating antioxidant responses for different plant species contaminated with heavy metals. The inhibition of catalase activity is essential for avoidance of heavy metal stress-related damage (Willekens et. al., 1995).

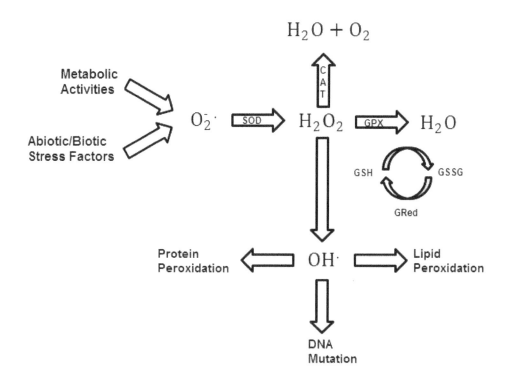

Fig. 1. Effects and results of ROS (Reactive Oxygen Species) (www.biozentrum.uni-frankfurt.de/Pharmakologie/index.html, 2008).

3. Detection of injury related to heavy metal accumulation in plants by molecular markers

With the invention of polymerase chain reaction (PCR) technology (Mullis & Faloona, 1987), PCR based molecular markers techniques were developed. Random amplified Polymorphic DNA (RAPD), one of the PCR based molecular marker techniques, is simple, rapid and low cost assay. The knowledge of genome is not required; in addition a single short random oligonucleotide primer is used. RAPD assay detects wide range of DNA damages (point mutations, inversions, deletions) and at the same time large number of samples can be studied. RAPD does not require radiolabelling for visualisation. In RAPD studies, similarities and diversities are described by appearance of new bands, disappearance of bands, and variation in band intensities. Despite its many advantages there are also some limitations. Generally it is claimed that RAPD profiles are not reproduciple but no evidence of such event is presented (Atienzar & Jha, 2006). After optimisation of RAPD, many studies have confirmed the reproducibility of the assay (Benter et. al., 1995; Atienzar et al., 2000).

Ecotoxicological literature displayed that RAPD assay is a fundamental tool to evaluate the effects of toxicants on organisms under optimized conditions. For genetoxicity studies, RAPD can be used as a diagnostic marker. The presence, absence and intensity of bands are related to DNA damages, mutations by genotoxicants. RAPD assay was successfully used to monitorize DNA changes induced by heavy metals such as lead, cadmium, copper (Enan, 2006; Liu et al., 2005; Körpe and Aras, 2011), UV and x-ray (Kuroda et al., 1999). DNA changes include damages and mutations that can be generated by toxicants directly and/or indirectly. According to RAPD profile, the genomic template stability (GTS, %) could be calculated as '100 – (100 (a/n))' where 'n' is the number of bands in control RAPD profile and 'a' the average number of changes in sample profiles. DNA damages and mutations may alter a primer binding site and thus genomic template stability changes and polymorphism occurs within dose-dependent treatments and non-treatment organisms.

The toxic effects of heavy metals on plants can be detected with various biomarkers. The use of both population and molecular marker is fundamental to determine clearly the effects of toxicants on organisms. Liu et al. (2005) used barley (*Hordeum vulgare* L.) seedlings as bioindicator of cadmium pollution, changes were observed by total soluble protein level, root growth as population markers and RAPD as molecular marker. In another study, rice (*Oryza sativa* L.) seedlings were exposed to Cd concentrations. To assess the effects of Cd on plants; growth parameters, levels of gluthatione and phytochelatins were measured and Amplified Fragment Length Polymorphism (AFLP) technique was used to determine the Cd induced genetic variation (Aina et al., 2007).

AFLP is a method generated by restriction digestion of genomic DNA, ligation of adapters (recognition sequences to restricted DNA), pre amplification reactions, selective amplification, gel electrophoresis (polyacrylamide gel), followed by visualization through autoradiography or by fluorescence methods. In AFLP assay, the number of selective nucleotides in AFLP primers, motif of selective nucleotide and genome size (Agarwall et al., 2008). AFLP assay does not require any prior knowledge of DNA sequence. AFLP assay is a successful tool for measuring genotoxic activity due to toxicants. In heavy metal polluted and nonpolluted areas, Muller et al. (2004) described genetic variation of *Suillus luteus* population using AFLP In other study, *Arabidopsis thaliana* (L.) was used as bioindicators of two genotoxic substances (potassium dichromate and dihydrophenanthrene) (Labra et al., 2003). To evaluate the effects of organic and inorganic genotoxic substances, germination test and AFLP analysis were used.

Eggplant (*Solanum melongena* L.) seedlings as bioindicator of a range of copper concentrations were studied with population and molecular markers in our laboratory (Körpe and Aras, 2011). Treated and non-treated groups were analysed, changes in growth were detected with root lenght, dry weight, total soluble protein content and changes in DNA with RAPD assay. Root-biomass production was significantly decreased by increased Cu^{2+} concentrations ($P < 0.05$) after 21 days of exposure, compared with the control seedlings. The principal events observed following the exposure to Cu^{2+} were the loss of normal bands and appearance of new bands, compared with the normal control seedlings. We found that these changes were dose-dependent. The use of various biomarkers could help to detect the effects of toxicants at various levels of the organism's health status (Liu et al., 2007).

Cu^{2+} and Zn^{2+} participate in vital growth processes such as mineral nutrition, photosynthesis, mitochondrial respiration, cell wall metabolism and hormone signaling pathways (Nussbaum et al., 1988; Costa de et. al., 1994). Soydam Aydın et. al., (2011a in process); compared the effects of Cu^{2+}, Zn^{2+} and $Cu^{2+}+Zn^{2+}$ treatments on root elongation, dry weight, total protein and changes in RAPD band profiles of cucumber (*Cucumis sativus* L.). As a result, cumulative and antagonistic effect were observed between Cu^{2+} and Zn^{2+} contamination in terms of population parameters and RAPD band profiles. It was shown that root lengths of cucumber were decreased with the increased concentration ($p<0.01$) of Cu^{2+}, Zn^{2+} and $Cu^{2+}+Zn^{2+}$ treatments after 21d of exposure. Authors suggested that DNA damages and mutations might alter primer binding sites and thus genomic template stability changes due to metal exposure are shown in Table 1. GTS values belong to Cu contaminations were approximately conserved at 40-45 % levels. Generally, lower GTS values were observed at the lower concentrations of metals. Effects of combined solutions were higher than the effects Cu^{2+} alone on GTS values (Table 1). An extreme adverse affect was observed at all concentrations of Zn^{2+} treatments which the effects of Zn^{+2} treatment on DNA remained to be identified.

Tomato (*Lycopersicon esculentum* L.) seeds germinated in various concentrations of $Pb(NO_3)_2$ solution were used for measuring population parameters such as dry weight, total soluble protein content, radicula length and ultimately in IRs and also determining genotoxic effect of lead reflecting as appearance or disappearance of bands in RAPD profiles in our laboratory. Inhibition or activation of radicula elongation was considered to be the first evident effect of metal toxicity in the tested plants. The data obtained from RAPD band profiles and GTS revealed consistent results with the population parameters especially total soluble protein content. There was a positive correlation between GTS values and root growth results (dry weight, radicula length) at 40 ppm Pb^{+2} contaminated samples. On the other hand, 40 ppm was considered as the point of maximum appearance and disappearance of new bands in RAPD assay (Table 2).

Because of high reactivity of Cd^{+2}, it can directly influence growth, senescence and energy synthesis processes (Tiquia et. al., 1996; Turner et.al., 2002). Cadmium (Cd^{+2}) is a multitarget toxicant for most organisms studied, and it is a well established human carcinogen. DNA damage induced by Cd^{+2} contamination has been shown by changes in RAPD profile (disappearance of bands and appearance of new PCR products occured in the profiles) compared with root elongation, dry weight, total protein amount (Soydam Aydın et. al., 2011b in press). Changes in the soluble protein content of root tips in okra seedlings exhibited a significant decrease with the increased concentration of Cd^{+2} contamination. Most of the new band appearances and disappearances in RAPD assay were shown in 30 ppm contamination which maximum inhibition of total protein contenthas also occured. This research concluded that Cd has a genotoxic effect which may induce DNA mutation or structural changes and RAPD is a suitable molecular marker for screening DNA damage induced by non-lethal levels of Cd solutions. Effect of different heavy metal concentrations on RAPD profiles reflect as changes in GTS (%). According to comparison of GTS % between plant and heavy metal, the most stabile genomic template was determined in tomato seedlings exposed to 80 ppm and 240 ppm Pb^{+2} concentrations. The most significant reduction was seen at 640 ppm Zn^{2+} solution and a direct proportion was found in this metal concentration with GTS values, root length and dry weight in cucumber seedlings. It was remarkable that different concentrations of Zn^{2+} significantly decreased average GTS (%) values in cucumber, while GTS values of Pb exposed tomato seedlings were average at 85,55 %. We determined heavy metal toxicity on higher plants and on the basis of GTS % inhibition and they showed the following order: Zn > Cu >Cd Pb > (Figure 2.).

Heavy metal Concentration	Averange % GTS values of Cu exposed eggplant	Averange % GTS values of Pb exposed tomato	Average %GTS values of Cd exposed okra	Average %GTS values of Cu^{2+} exposed cucumber	Average %GTS values of Zn^{2+} exposed cucumber	Average %GTS values of combined solution of Cu^{2+} Zn^{2+} exposed cucumber
Control	100	100	100	100	100	100
30 ppm	90	-	59.0	-	-	-
40 ppm	-	78,14	-	40,85	2,56	15,98
60 ppm	77,5	-	76,4	-		
80 ppm	-	90,62	-	41,54	7,62	15,98
120 ppm	53,75	81,81	72.5	-	-	-
160 ppm	-	87,10	-	45,76	7,62	30,69
240 ppm	46,25	90,08	-	45,90	4,44	42,05
320 ppm	-	-	-	51,27	1,58	35,02
640 ppm	-	-	-	29,40	1,95	38,69

(-) Not recorded

Table 1. Effect of different heavy metals concentration on GTS of plant.

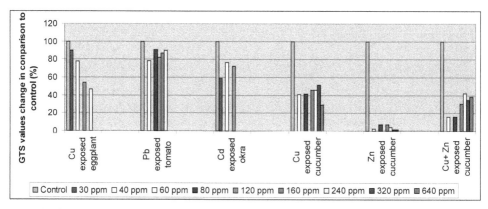

Fig. 2. % change in GTS values in comparison to control.

4. Detection of injury related with heavy metal accumulation in plants by real-time PCR

Before using real- time PCR to detect heavy metal injury in plants, the first question is what is the real time PCR? Some believe the growth of the amplification curves have to be able to watch during PCR on a computer monitor in order to be truly 'real-time'. This of course is not the case but is not the only reason for using real-time PCR. It has many advantages when compared with conventional PCR system. While conventional PCR systems have many disadvantages as labor intense, hazardous materials (e.g., 32P), low resolution & sensitivity, low dynamic range, poor discrimination among homologous genes or transcript sizes, results not expressed as numbers, not very quantitative, real-time PCR solve all these problems (Dorak, 2006). A PCR reaction has three phases, exponential phase, linear phase and plateau phase as conventional PCR and during the exponential phase PCR product will ideally double during each cycle if efficiency is perfect, i.e. 100% (Joshua et al., 2006).

The major disadvantages of real-time PCR are that it requires expensive equipment and reagents. In addition, due to its extremely high sensitivity, hard experimental design and an in-depth understanding of normalization techniques are imperative for accurate conclusions (Marisa et al., 2005). Data should be normalized absolutely or relatively. Absolute quantification employs an internal or external calibration curve to derive the input template copy number.The standard or calibration curve which we generated with Light Cycler 480 real-time PCR instrument is shown in Figure 3. Absolute quantification is important in case that the exact transcript copy number needs to be determined, while, relative quantification is sufficient for most physiological and pathological studies. Relative quantification relies on the comparison between expression of a target gene versus a reference gene and the expression of same gene in target sample versus reference samples (Pfaffl, 2001).

Attia et. al., 2009 used quantitaive real- time PCR to determine the regulation of superoxide dismutase gene expression under light conditions interacts with salt stress in *Arabidopsis thaliana* plants (Col, Columbia, and N1438). Plants were grown for 15 d under two light regimes provides different growth rates. The medium contained 0–85 mM NaCl. Shoot biomass and ion accumulation were measured. Superoxide dismutase (SOD) activity was assayed on gels, and the expressions of SOD genes were studied using real-time PCR.

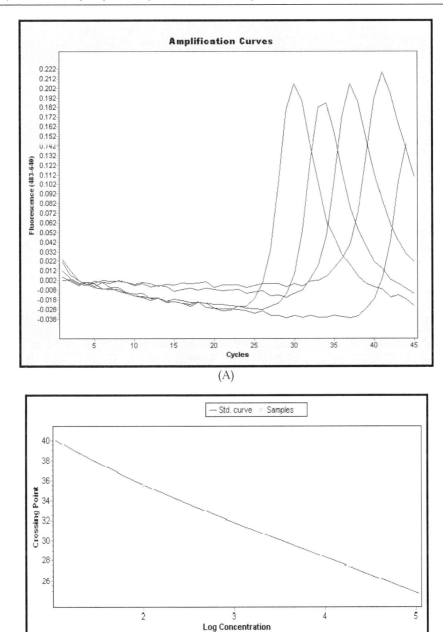

(A)

(B)

Fig. 3. Real-time PCR. (A) The PCR amplification curve charts the accumulation of fluorescent emission at each reaction cycles of standart curve.(B) is the output of a serial dilution experiment from an Light Cycler 480 real-time PCR instrument (Efficiency: 1.937 Error: 0.00769 Slope: -3.483 YIntercept: 43.43)

Research hypothesizing that oxidative stress occurred when light energy input exceeded energy utilization when salt inhibited growth, and that oxidative stress induced overexpression of some SOD genes.

The molecular responses of hydroponically cultivated tomato plants to As(V) or Cr(VI) were assessed by transcript accumulation analysis of genes coding for products potentially involved in heavy metal tolerance. A quantitative real-time PCR experiment was performed to determine the effects of As(V) or Cr(VI) at concentrations ranging from 80 to 640 mM on protein genes Hsp90-1, MT2- and GR1-like using RNA isolated from 24h treated tomato roots or shoots. As(V) increased MT2- and GR1-like transcripts in treated tomato roots but Cr(VI) treatment slightly affected the transcript levels (Goupila et. al., 2009).

A quantitative real-time PCR assay was used to determine transgene copy number in some plants and one of the most sensitive and reliably quantitative methods for gene expression analysis (Chiang et al., 1996; Ingham et al., 2001; Callaway et al., 2002; Song et al., 2002). Many researchers declare that, there is also need to know that what extent heavy metals can induce changes in major lipid components of the cell membranes. Most of these reports have been focused mainly on lipid peroxidation which induce production of ROS and represent the first targets for metal toxicity in plants (Somashekaraiah et. al., 1992; De Vos et al., 1993, Meharg, 1993).

Cd and Pb stress are shown to distrupt the cellular homeostasis and cause oxidative damage to plants due to increased level of reactive oxygen species (ROS) which cause lipid peroxidation, membrane defects and unstability of enzymes in higher plants. Based on the knowledge of ROS a study was conducted to determine the effects of lead (Pb) and cadmium (Cd) elements on lipid peroxidation, catalase enzyme activity and gene expression profile in tomato (*Lycopersicum esculentum* L.). 25 days-old plants grown in controlled media were used for stress treatments. For application of heavy metal stress Pb and Cd were added to the hydroponic solution for 24h at a concentration from 0 (control), 80, 160, 320, 640 and 1280 mM of Pb or Cd.

Estimation of lipid peroxidation analysis based malondialdehyde (MDA) which is a marker of oxidative lipid injury which changes in response to environmental factors lead to stress in plants (Hodges et.al., 1999) and the most significant increase in the MDA content were seen in the samples exposed to 320 µM concentration of Pb contamination, while the lowest degree of MDA content was determined at the samples exposed to 1280 µM concentration of Pb. Assay of catalase activity was performed by the method of Aebi et. al., (1988) based on 240 nm absorbance and quantitative real-time PCR was performed with Light Cycler ® 480 System (Roche), thermal cycler. Primers and probes sequences (presented in Table 2) of target gene catalase (CAT) and actin (ACT) used for normalization were designated on sequences of tomato genes available in the databank (http://www.ncbi.nlm. nih.gov/).

CAT gene expressions showed a complex pattern under heavy metal contamination and enzyme activity results were strongly up-regulated with this pattern at the same concentration ($p<0.05$). Our results confirm that heavy metal contaminations are related to impairment of ETS (Electron transport system) of membranes that caused an increase of forms of reactive oxygen species (ROS) includes O_2^-, H_2O_2, OH^- and HO^{2-}. Many genes play a crucial role for responding heavy metal stresses at transcriptional level and CAT is one of these genes that encode catalase enzyme. In this case, CAT as an antioxidant defense system

CAT2 F	CTTTCCTCTTCgACgATATTggTA
CAT2 S	TATTCCCCAAgATTACAggCAT
CAT2 A	CCgACTCggATTgCCTT
CAT2 R	gTgATTTgCTCCTCCgACTC
CAT2 FL	CAACAgggCTggAAAATCAACTTATgT-FL
CAT2 LC 640	AAgTTCCACTggAAgCCCACATgT p
ACT F	CATTgTCCACAgAAAgTgCTTCTA
ACT S	TCTgTTTCCCggTTTTgCTATTAT
ACT A	AACCACATTAAATggAAACATgAgAT
ACT R	TgCATCAggCACCTCTCAAg
Actin FL	ATTCATAgCCCCCACCACCAAAC-FL
Actin LC 640	TCTCCATCCCATCAAAAAAACAAATTgACT p

Table 2. Primer and Probe Sequences of CAT (catalase) and ACT (actin).

component, which can protect plants from cellular injury by removing excessively produced H_2O_2, is activated (Qilin et al., 2009).

5. Conclusion

The results of these studies have shown the advantages of using plants as bioindicator of heavy metal toxicity. Plants could develop different defense mechanisms against heavy metal stress such as storing toxic metals in roots in order to prevent the dispersal of ions into the other parts of the plant (Fernandes & Henriques, 1991). Also, alteration in total soluble protein content is one of the important effect which promote senescence or reduce protein synthesis by preventing the protein content of plants (Gupta, 1986). To measure of some parameters at the population level can facilitate the interpretation of the data at the molecular level. Though the plant genome is very stable, its DNA might be damaged due to the exposure to stress factors and it can be shown as differences in band profiles of molecular markers. Plants exposed to heavy metal stress also show rapid and temporary drops in growth rate and activate antioxidant defense system by producing ROS which alter MDA content and gene expression and enzyme activity patterns of CAT. We also suggest that; molecular markers such as RAPD, AFLP combined with population biomarker and quantitative real-time PCR technique can be used for determining the effects of heavy metal toxicity in plants and real –time PCR is the most reliable technique to determine the responses given by the plant against heavy metal toxicity at gene expression level.

6. Acknowledgement

The authors would like to thank to Ankara University Biotechnology Institute for providing the real time PCR equipment for the studies. The authors would also like to thank to Ankara University Biotechnology Institute for the partial support of the other equipments by the projects number 61 and 171.

7. References

Aebi, C.; Lafontaine, E.R., Cope, L.D., Latimer, J.L., Lumbley, S.L., McCracken, G.H.,Jr & Hansen, E.J. (1998). Phenotypic effect of isogenic *uspA*1 and *uspA*2 mutations on *Moraxella catarrhalis* O35E. Infection and Immunity, Vol. 66, pp. 3113–3119

Agarwall, M.; Shrivastava, N. & Padh, H. (2008). Advances in molecular marker techniques and their applications in plant sciences. *Plant Cell Reports*, Vol. 27, No. 4, pp. 617-631

Aina, R.; Labra, M., Fumagalli, P., Vannini, C., Marsoni, M., Cucchi, U., Bracale, M., Sgorbati, S. & Citterio, S. (2007). Thiol-peptide level and proteomic changes in response to cadmium toxicity in *Oryza sativa* L. roots. *Environmental and Experimental Botany*, Vol. 59, No. 3, pp. 381-892

Alirzayeva, E. G.; Shirvani, T. S., Yazici, M. A., Alverdiyeva, S., M., Shukurov, E. S., Ozturk, L., Ali-Zade, V. M. & Cakmak, I. (2006). Heavy metal accumulation in Artemisia and foliaceous lichen species from the Azerbaijan flora. *Forest Snow and Landscape Research*, Vol. 80, No. 3, pp. 339-348

Angelone, M. & Bini C. (1992). Trace element concentrations in soils and plants of Western Europe. In: Adriano DC (Ed.). Biogeochemistry of trace elements, CRC Press, Boca Raton, FL: Levis Publishers pp. 19-60

Arnon, D. I. & Stout, P. R. (1939). The essentiality of certain elements in minute quantity for plants with special reference to copper. *Plant Physiology*, Vol. 14, pp. 371-375,

Asada, K. (2006). Production and scavenging of reactive oxygen species in chloroplasts and their functions. *Plant Physiology*. Vol. 141; pp. 391–396.

Atienzar, F., Evenden, A., Jha, A., Savva, D., Depledge, M. (2000). Optimized RAPD analysis generates high-quality genomic DNA profiles at high annealing temperature. *Biotechniques*, Vol. 28, No. 1, pp. 52-54,

Atienzar, F.A., Jha, A.N. (2006). The random amplified polymorphic DNA (RAPD) assay and related techniques applied to genotoxicity and carcinogenesis studies: a critical review. *Mutation Research*, Vol. 613, No. 2-3, pp. 76-102

Attia, H.;F Karray, N. & Lachaâl M. (2009). Light interacts with salt stress in regulating superoxide dismutase gene expression in Arabidopsis *Plant Science* Vol.177, pp. 161–167

Aust, S. D., Morehouse, L. A. & Thomas, C. E. (1985). Role of metals in oxygen radical reactions. *Free Radicals Biology and Medicine*. Vol. 1, pp. 3-25

Baccini, P. (1985). Metal transport and metalbiota interaction in lakes. *Environmental Technology Letters*, Vol. 6, pp. 327–334.

Baker, E. L.; Peterson, W. A., Holtz, J. L. Coleman, C., & Landrigan, P. J. (1979). Subacute Cadmium Intoxication in Jewelry Workers: An Evaluation of Diagnostic Procedures. *Archives of Environmental Health*, Vol. 34, pp. 173-177

Becana M.; Dalton D.A., Moran J.F., Iturbe-Ormaetxe I, Matamoros M.A., & Rubio M.C. (2000). Reactive oxygen species and antioxidants in legume nodules. *Physiologia Plantatum*. 109: 372–381.

Benter, T.; Papadopoulos, S., Pape, M., Manns, M. & Poliwoda, H. (1995). Optimization and reproducibility of random amplified polymorphic DNA in human. *Analytical Biochemistry*, Vol. 230, No. 1, pp. 92-100

Boussama, N.; Ouariti, O. & Ghorbel, M.H. (1999a). Changes in growth and nitrogen assimilation in barley seedlings under cadmium stress. *Journal of Plant Nutrition*, Vol. 22, pp. 731–752

Boussama, N.; Ouariti, O., Suzuki, A. & Ghorbal, M.H. (1999b). Cd stress on nitrogen assimilation. *Journal of Plant Physiology*, Vol. 155, pp. 310–317

Callaway A.S.; Abranches R., Scroggs J., Allen G.C., & Thompson W.F. (2002). High throughput transgene copy number estimation by competitive PCR. *Plant Molecular Biology Reporter*. Vol. 20, pp. 265-277.

Chaney, R.L. (1993). Zinc phytotoxicity. In: Robson AD, ed. Zinc in soils and plants. Dordrecht, The Netherlands: *Kluwer Academic Publishers*, pp. 135-150.

Chaudhry N & Qurat-ul-Ain Y, (2003), Effect of Growth Hormones i.e., IAA, Kinetin and Heavy Metal i.e., Lead Nitrate on the Internal Morphology of Leaf of Phaseolus vulgaris L. *Pakistan Journal of Biological Sciences*, Vol. 6;2, pp 157-163.

Chiang, P.W.; Song WJ, Wu KY, Korenberg JR, Fogel EJ, Van Keuren ML, Lashkari D, and Kurnit DM. (1996). Use of a fluorescent-PCR reaction to detect genomic sequence copy number and transcriptional abundance. *Genome Research*, Vol. 6, pp. 1013-1026

Constantine, M.J. & Owens, E.T. (1982). Introduction and Perspectives of Plant Genetic and Cytogenetic Assays: A Report of the U.S. Environmental Protection Agency Gene-Tox Program, *Mutation Research*, Vol. 99, pp 1-12

Costa de, C.A.; Casali, V.W.D., Loures, E.G., Cecon, P.R., Jordão, C.P. (1994). Content level of heavy metals in lettuce (*Lactuca sativa* L.) fertilized with organic compost from urban waste. *Revista Ceres*, Vol. 238, pp. 629–640

De Vos, C.H.R.; Ten Boukum W.M., Vooijs, R., Schar H. & De Kok, L.J. (1993). Effect of copper on fatty acid composition and peroxidaiton of lipids in the roots of copper tolerant and sensitive *Silene cucbalus. Plant Physiology Biochemistry*, Vol. 31, pp. 151-158

Del Rı́o, L.A, Lyon S., Olah I., Glick B, & Salin, M.L. (1983) Immunocytochemical evidence for a peroxisomal localization of manganese superoxide dismutase in leaf protoplasts from a higher plant. *Planta*, Vol. 158, pp. 216–224

Doncheva, S.; Nikolov, B. & Ogneva, V. (1996). Effect of excess copper on the morphology of the nucleus in maize root meristem cells. *Physiologia Plantarum*, Vol. 96 (1), pp. 118-122

Dong, J.; Wu, F., Zhang, G. (2006). Influence of cadmium on antioxidant capacity and four microelement concentrations in tomato seedlings (*Lycopersicon esculentum*). *Chemosphere*, Vol. 64, pp. 1659–1666

Dorak, T. (2006). Real-Time PCR. An introduction to real-time PCR Taylor & Francis Group. http://www.gene-quantification.de

Droillard M.J. & Paulin A. (1990). Isozymes of superoxide dismutase in mitochondria and in peroxisomes isolated from petals of carnation during senescence. *Plant Physiology*, Vol. 94, pp. 1187-1192.

Enan, M.R. (2006). Application of random amplified polymorphic DNA (RAPD) to detect the genotoxic effect of heavy metals. *Biotechnology and Applied Biochemistry*, Vol. 43, No. 3, pp. 147-154

Florijn, P.J., &Van Beusichem, M.L. (1993). Uptake and distribution of cadmium in maize inbred lines. *Plant and Soil*, Vol. 150, pp. 25-32

Freedman, B., & Hutchinsotn, C. (1980). Effects of smelter pollutants on forest leaf litter decomposition near a nickel-copper smelter at Sudbury, Ontario. *Canadian Journal of Botany*,Vol. 58, pp. 1722-1736

Freedman, B. & Hutchinson, T.C. (1981). Sources of metal and elemental contaminants of terrestrial environments. In: Lepp NW, editor. Effect of heavy metal pollution on plants: Metals in the environment, London and New Jersey: *Applied Science Publishers*, Vol. 11, pp. 35-94

Fernandes, J. C. & Henriques, F.S., (1991). Biochemical, physiological and structural effect of excess copper in plants, *The Botanical Review*, Vol. 57, pp. 246-273.

Fridovich, I. (1995) Superoxide radical and superoxide dismutases. *Annual Review Biochemistry*, Vol. 64, pp. 97–112.

Grant, W.F. (1994). The present status of higher plant bioassays for the detection of environmental mutagens. *Mutation Research* Vol. 310, pp. 175-185

Greger, M. & Lindberg, S. (1987). Effects of Cd^{2+} and EDTA on young sugar beets (Beta vulgaris). I. Cd^{2+} uptake and sugar accumulation. *Physiologia Plantarum*, Vol. 66, pp. 69-74

Goupila, P.; Souguira,D., Ferjanib, E., Faurec, O., Hitmid, A. & Ledoigta, G. (2009). Expression of stress-related genes in tomato plants exposed to arsenic and chromium in nutrient solution. *Journal of Plant Physiology*. Vol. 166(13:1), pp. 1446-1452

Gupta, U.C. (1979). Boron nutrition of crops. *Advances in Agronomy*, Vol. 31, pp. 273-307

Gupta, S.L. (1986). Copper uptake and inhibition of growth, photosynthetic pigments and macromolecules in the cyanobacterium Anacystis nidulans. *Photosynthetica*. Vol. 20 (4), pp. 447-453

Halliwell, B. & Gutteridge, J.M.C. (1989). Protection against oxidants in biological systems: The superoxide theory of oxygen toxicity. In: Halliwell, B., Gutteridge, J.M.C. (Eds) Free radicals in biology and medicine. *Clarendon Press*, Oxford.

Hodges, D.M.; DeLong J.M., Forney C.F. & Prange, R.K. (1999). Improving the thiobarbituric acid reactive substances assay for estimating lipid peroxidation in plant tissues containing anthocyanin and other interfering compounds. *Planta*, Vol. 207, pp. 604–611

Humphrey, M. O., & Nicholls, M. K. (1984). Relationships between tolerance to heavy metals in Agrostis cupillaris L. (*A. tenuis* Sibth.). *New Phytology*, Vol. 98, pp. 177-190

Ingham D.J.; Beer S, Money S., & Hansen G. (2001) Quantitative real-time PCR assay for determining transgene copy number in transformed plants. *Biotechniques*, Vol. 31, pp. 132-134, 136-140

Jimi, E.; Aoki, K., Saito H., D'Acquisto, F., May, M.J. & Nakamura, I. (2004). Selective inhibition of NF-kappa B blocks osteoclasto-genesis and prevents inflammatory bone destruction in vivo. *Nature Medicine*, Vol. 10, pp. 617–624

Joshua S. Y.; Reed, A., Chen, F. & Neal Stewart, C. (2006). Statistical analysis of real-time PCR data. *BMC Bioinformatics*. Methodology article.

Kachenko, A. & Singh, B. (2004). Heavy metals contamination of home grown vegetables near smelters in NSW. SuperSoil: *3rd Australian New Zealand Soils Conference*, 5-9 December 2004, University of Sydney, Australia

Kanazawa, T.; Nakamura, S. Momoi, M. Yamaji, T. Takematsu, H. Yano, H. Sabe, H., Yamamoto, A., Kawasaki, T. & Kozutsumi, Y. (2000). Inhibition of cytokinesis by a lipid metabolite, psychosine. *The Journal of Cell Biology*, Vol. 149, pp. 943–950

Kılıç, Z.; Dönmez Ç., Soydam Aydın, & S., Aras, S. (2011). Monitoring the genotoxic effect of heavy metal pollution in tomato (*Lycopersicum esculentum* L.) by linking RAPD assay and population markers (in press).

Knasmuller, S., Gottmann, E., Steinkellner, H., Fomin, A., Pickl, C., God, R. & Kundi, M. (1998). Detection of genotoxic effects of heavy metal contaminated soils with plant bioassays. *Mutation Research*. Vol. 420, pp. 37-48

Körpe, D.A. & Aras, S. (2011). Evaluation of copper-induced stress on eggplant (*Solanum melongena* L.) seedlings at the molecular and population levels by use of various biomarkers. *Mutation Research*. Vol. 719, No. 1-2, pp. 29-34

Kuroda, S.; Yano, H., Koga-Ban, Y., Tabei, Y., Takaiwa, F., Kayano, T. & Tanaka, H. (1999). Identification of DNA polymorphism induced by X-ray and UV irradiation in plant cells. *Japan Agricultural Research Quarterly*, Vol. 33, pp. 223-226.

Labra, M.; Di Fabio, T., Grassi, F., Regondi, S.M., Bracale, M., Vannini, C. & Agradi, E. (2003). AFLP analysis as biomarker of exposure to organic and inorganic genotoxic substances in plants. *Chemosphere*. Vol. 52, No. 7, pp. 1183-1188

Li, X., Lin, H., Zhang, W., Zou, Y., Zhang, J., Tang, X. & Zhou, J.M. (2005). Flagellin induces innate immunity in nonhost interactions that is suppressed by Pseudomonas syringae effectors. *Proceedings of the National Academy of Sciences of the United States of America*, Vol. 102, pp. 12990-12995

Lidon, F.C. & Henriques F.S. (1991). Effects of copper on the ascorbate, diamine and O-diphenol oxidases activities of rice leaves. *Oyton-International Journal of Experimental Botany*, Vol. 52, pp. 97–104

Lin, C.C. & Kao, C.H. (1999). NaCl induced changes in ionically bound peroxidase activity in roots of rice seedlings. *Plant and Soil*, Vol. 216, pp. 147-153

Lin, C.C. & Kao, C.H. (2000). Effect of NaCl stress on H_2O_2 metabolism in rice leaves. *Plant Growth Regulation*, Vol. 30, pp. 151-155

Lipman, C.B., & McKinney, G. (1931). Proof of the essential nature of copper for higher green plants. *Plant Physiology*, Vol. 6, pp. 539–599.

Liu, W.; Li, P., Qi, X.M., Zhou, Q., Zheng, L., Sun, T., Yang, Y. (2005). DNA changes in barley (*Hordeum vulgare*) seedlings induced by cadmium pollution using RAPD analysis. *Chemosphere*, Vol. 61, pp. 158-167

Liu, W.; Yang, Y.S., Zhou, Q., Xie, L., Li, P., Sun, T. (2007). Impact assessment of cadmiumcontamination on rice (*Oryza sativa* L.) seedlings at molecular and populationlevels using multiple biomarkers. *Chemosphere*, Vol. 67 (6), pp. 1155-1163

Marisa, L.; Wong, J. F. & Medrano (2005) Real-time PCR for mRNA quantitation. *BioTechniques*. Vol. 39, pp. 75-85.

Mazé, P. (1915). Détermination des éléments minéraux rares nécessaires au développement du maïs. *Comptes Rendus Hebdomadaires des Séances de L'académie des Sciences*, Vol. 160, pp. 211–214

Meharg, A.A. (1993). The role of the plasmalemma in metal tolerance in angiosperms. *Physiologica Plantarum*, Vol. 88, pp. 191-198

McCord, J.M. & Fridovich, I. (1969). Superoxide dismutase: an enzymic function for erythrocuprein (hemocuprein). *The Journal of Biological Chemistry*, Vol. 244, pp. 6049-55

Miller, A.F. &. Sorkin D.L (1997) "Superoxide Dismutases: A Molecular Perspective" *Comments on Molecular and Cellular Biophysics*, Vol. 9(1), pp. 1 - 48

Moore, J.W. & Ramamoorthy, S. (1984). Heavy metals in natural waters. *Springer Verlag*, New York, USA, pp. 268

Moustakas, M.; Lanaras, T., Symeonidis, L. & Karataglis, S. (1994). Growth and some photosynthetic characteristics of field grown *Avena sativa* under copper and lead stress. *Photosynthetica*, Vol. 30, pp. 389-396

Muller, L.A.H.; Lambaerts, M., Vangronsveld J., Colpaert, V. (2004). AFLP-based assessment of the effects of environmental heavy metal pollution on the genetic structure of pioneer populations of *Suillus luteus*. *New Phytologist*, Vol. 164, pp. 297-303.

Mullis, K.B. & Faloona, F.A. (1987). Specific synthesis of DNA in vitro via a polymerase-catalyzed chain reaction. *Methods in Enzymology*, Vol. 155, pp. 335-350

Munzuroglu, O. & Geckil, H. (2002). Effects of metals on seed germination, root elongation, and coleoptile and hypocotyl growth in *Triticum aestivum* and *Cucumis sativus*. *Archives Environmental Contamination and Toxicology*, Vol. 43, pp. 203–213

Nedelkoska, T.V. & Doran, P.M. (2000), Characteristics of heavy metal uptake by plant species with potential for phytoremediation and phytomining, *Minerals Engineering*, Vol. 13, pp. 549-561

Nriagu, J.O., (1978). Biogeochemistry Of Lead In The Environment. *Elsevier Biomedical Press*, Amsterdam, Vol. 1, pp. 422, Vol. 2, pp. 379

Nriagu, J.O. (1979). The global copper cycle. Copper in the environment. Part 1: Ecological Cycling. John Wiley, NY. Vol. 1, pp. 1-7

Nussbaum S.; Schmutz D & Brunold C. (1988) Regulation of assimilatory sulfate reduction by cadmium in *Zea mays* L. *Plant Physiology*, Vol. 88, pp. 1407-1410

Ouzounidou, G.; Eleftheriou E.P. & Karataglis S. (1992). Ecophysiological and ultrastructural effects of copper in *Thlaspi ochroleucum* (Curciferae). *Canadian Journal of Botany.*, Vol. 70, pp. 947–957

Patra, G.; Vaissaire, J., Weber-Levy, M., Le Doujet, C. & Mock, M. (1998). Molecular characterisation of Bacillus strains involved in outbreaks of anthrax in France in 1997. *Journal of Clinical Microbiology*, Vol. 36, pp. 3412–3414

Pfaffl M.W. (2001). A new mathematical model for relative quantificationin real-time RT-PCR. Nucleic Acids Research. Vol. 29, pp. 2002-2007

Poschenrieder, C.; Gunsé, B. & Barceló, J. (1989). Influence of cadmium on water relations, stomatal resitance, and abscisic acid content in expanding bean leaves. *Plant Physiology*. Vol. 90, pp. 1465-1371

Rai, L.C. & Raizada, M. (1988). Impact of chromium and lead on Nostoc muscorum: Regulation of toxicity by ascorbic acid, glutathione and sulphur-containing amino acids. *Ecotoxicology and Environmental Safety*, Vol. 15, pp. 195-205

Salin, M.L. & Bridges, S.M. (1980). Isolation and characterization of an iron-containing superoxide dismutase from a eucaryote, *Brassica campestris*. *Archives of Biochemistry and Biophysics*, Vol. 201, pp. 369-374

Sandermann, H.J.R. (1994). Higher plant metabolism of xenobiotics: the 'green liver' concept. *Pharmacogenetics*. Vol. 4(5), pp. 225–241

Salomons, W., & Forstner, U. (1984) Metals in the hydrocycle. Springer-Verlag, Berlin, Heidelberg, New York, Tokyo.

Sandalio, L.M.; Dalurzo, H.C., Gomes, M., Romero-Puertas, M. & Del Rio, L.A. (2001). Cadmium- induced changes in the growth and oxidative metabolism of pea plants. *Journal of Experimental Botany*, Vol. 52, pp. 2115-2126

Shah, K. & Dubey, R.S. (1995). Cadmium induced changes on germination, RNA level and ribonuclease activity in rice seeds. *Plant Physiology and Biochemistry (India)*. Vol. 22, pp. 101-107

Sharma, P. &Dubey R.S. (2005). Lead toxicity in plants. *Brazilian Journal of Plant Physiology*, Vol.17, pp. 35-52

Skoog, F. (1940). Relationships between zinc and auxin in the growth of higher plants. *American Journal of Botany*, Vol. 27, pp. 939–951.

Song P.; Cai C.Q., Skokut M, Kosegi B.D., & Petolino J.F. (2002). Quantitative real-time PCR as a screening tool for estimating transgene copy number in WHISKERSTM derived transgenic maize. *Plant Cell Reports*. Vol. 20, pp. 948-954

Somashekaraiah, B.V.; Padmaja, K. & Prasad, A.R.K. (1992). Phytotoxicity of cadmium ions on germinating seedlings of mung bean (*Phaseolus vulgaris*): involvement of lipid peroxides in chlorophyll degradation. *Physiologia Plantarum*. Vol. 85, pp. 85-89

Sommer, A.L. & Lipman, C,B. (1926). Evidence on the indispensable nature of zinc and boron for higher green plants. *Plant Physiology*, Vol. 1, pp. 231–249

Sommer, A. L. (1931). Copper as an essential for plant growth. *Plant Physiology*, Vol. 6, pp. 339-345

Soydam Aydın, S.; Gökçe, E., Büyük, İ., Aras, S. (2011a) Characterization of Copper and Zinc induced stress on Cucumber (*Cucumis sativus* L.) by molecular and population parameters (in process *Mutation Research*)

Soydam Aydın, S.; Başaran, E., Cansaran-Duman, D., & Aras, S. (2011b). Genotoxic effect of cadmium in okra (*Abelmoschus esculantus* L.) seedlings: comperative inverstigation with population parameter and molecular marker.(in press).

Qadir, M.; Ghaffor, A., Murtaza, G. (2000). Cadmium concentration in vegetables grown on urban soils irrigated with untreated municipal sludge. *Environment Development Sustainability*, Vol. 2, pp. 11–19

Qilin, D., D. Wang Jin, W., Feng Bin, F., Liu Tingting, L., Chen Chen, C., Lin Honghui L., & Shizhang. D. (2009). Molecular cloning and characterization of a new peroxidase gene (OvRCI) from *Orychophragmus violaceus*. *African Journal of Biotechnology*. Vol. 8 (23), pp. 6511-6517

Tiquia, S. M., Tam, N. F. Y. & Hodgkiss, I. J. (1996). Effects of composting on phytotoxicity of spent pig-manure sawdust litter. *Environmental Pollution*. Vol. 93, pp. 249–256

Turner, J. G., Ellis, C. H., & Devoto, A. (2002). The jasmonate signal pathway. *Plant Cell*, Vol. 14(Suppl), pp. 153–164

Van Camp, W. (1994). Elevated levels of superoxide dismutase protect transgenic plants against ozone damage. *Biotechnology*, Vol. 12, pp. 165-168

Walsberg, M.; P. Joseph, B. Hale & Beyersmann, D. (2003). Molecular and cellular mechanisms of cadmium carcinogenesis. *Toxicology*, Vol. 192, pp. 95-117

Webber J., (1981) Trace metals in agriculture. In: N.W. Lepp (Ed.). Effect of heavy metal pollution on plants: Metals in the environment. Englewood: *Applied Science*. Vol. 2, pp: 159-184

Willekens,H.; Inze´,D., Van Montagu,M. & Van Camp,W. (1995). Catalases in plants. Mol. Breeding, 1, 207–228.

Yang, M.G.; Lin, X.Y., & Yang, X.E. (1998). Impact of Cd on growth and nutrient accumulation of different plant species. *Chinese Journal of Applied Ecology*, Vol. 19, pp. 89-94

Yi, T.H., & Ching, H.K. (2003). Changes in protein and amino acid contents in two cultivars of rice seedlings with different apparent tolerance to cadmium. *Plant Growth Regulation*, Vol. 40, pp. 147–155

Yoshida, Y. (2002). E3 ubiquitin ligase that recognizes sugar chains. *Nature*, Vol. 418, pp. 438–442

Zhou, Q.X. & Huang, G.H. (2001). Environmental Biogeochemistry and Global Environmental Changes (in Chinese). Beijing, China. *Science Press*, pp.144

Zhou, Q.X.; Cheng, Y., Zhang, Q.R., & Liang, J.D. (2003). Quantitative analyses of relationships between ecotoxicological effects and combined pollution. *Science in China Series C*. Vol. 33, pp. 566–573

http://www.ncbi.nlm. nih.gov/

www.biozentrum.uni-frankfurt.de/Pharmakologie/index.html, 2008

7

Genomic Sensitivity of Small Mammals - A Suitable Test System in the Genetic Monitoring

Margarita Topashka-Ancheva and Tsvetelina Gerasimova
Institute of Biodiversity and Ecosystem Research,
Bulgarian Academy of Sciences, Sofia
Bulgaria

1. Introduction

In recent decades, our attention is drawn to human-induced environmental changes and their potential threat to life on Earth through a growing number of mutagens and their effects on the biota. Genetic damage caused by these factors often have a durable effect that is manifested in later generations. The establishment of induced genetic damage in plants, animals and men is one of the most important issues in mutagenesis studies. With each passing year, the environment under anthropogenic influence is loaded with various toxicants. They affect living organisms directly, i.e. on the implementation of individual development, reducing the vitality of the individual, and hence - the population and the species as a whole. Not less important, although more discreetly, their impact remains on the inherited structures of the organisms. It is defined as mutagenic in the broadest sense.

Deleterious alterations in cellular DNA result from endogenous sources of damage as well as from external radiations and genotoxic chemicals in the environment. These alterations can cause mutations, genetic recombination, chromosomal aberrations, oncogenic processes or cell death. All genotoxic agents are capable to induce chromosomal aberrations efficiently (Natarajan, 1993). The types and the frequencies of aberrations induced depend upon the nature of agents, cell cycle stage treated and the cell type employed.

Genetic toxicology deals with the mutagenic effects of chemicals and radiation and reveals their mutagenicity on the biodiversity. Cytogenetic endpoints - chromosomal aberrations, sister chromatid exchanges, mitotic index and micronuclei have long been used to assess exposure of human populations to genotoxic agents. Chromosomal rearrangements are sensitive endpoint towards the action of genotoxins with various origins. Chromosomal aberrations are changes in chromosome structure, which involve gross alteration of the genetic material and are detected using light microscopy. Structural chromosomal aberrations may be induced mainly by direct DNA breakage, by replication on a damaged DNA template, and by inhibition of DNA synthesis (Sorsa et al., 1992; Albertini et al., 2000). They can be divided into two main classes: chromosome-type aberrations involving both chromatids of one or multiple chromosomes and chromatid-type aberrations involving only one of the two chromatids (Albertini et al., 2000; Hagmar et al., 2004). The application of cytogenetic observations is useful and informative approach in carefully controlled study designs concerning the risk assessment (Sorsa et al., 1990; Vanjo & Sorsa, 1991; Testa et al., 2002).

Cytogenetics offers a direct connection between mutagenicity tests in experimental organisms and effects in humans and is most often used in detecting human mutagen exposures (Bender et al., 1988; Sorsa et al., 1992). Chromosomal aberrations including chromatid breaks, chromatid exchanges, acentric fragments, dicentric chromosomes, ring chromosomes and some inversions and translocations can be reported in peripheral lymphocytes in people who have been exposed to mutagens. Increased frequencies of aberrations were found after exposure to ionizing radiation and various chemicals including benzene, cyclophosphamide, nickel containing compounds, vinyl chloride and styrene (Sorsa et al., 1992) and industrial polymetal dust (Topashka & Teodorova, 2010). Micronucleus formation results from breakage of chromatids or chromosomes when an acentric fragment is produced. Micronucleus test substitutes the metaphase analysis in human monitoring (Sorsa et al. 1992). Therefore, assays detecting chromosomal aberration or micronuclei are suitable for detecting genotoxic agents and clastogens (CSGMT, 1992).

Although all gathered evidences clearly showing the adverse effects of pollution on nature many people still remain unconcerned unless their own health is in danger. Human subjects would provide the most reliable information for risk assessment on human health and ecological risk, but this is not an accepted practice for many ethical reasons. Investigations which use suitable animal test systems and answers they could give may be a potential bridge to meet the gap between the animal-based and human-based environmental observations (O'Brien et al., 1993). The use of mammals to assess the human exposure to toxic environmental contaminants is unquestionable. Pet animals could provide valuable information of whether their owners are threatened by the contaminated environment. Reynolds et al (1994) have found evidence that absorption and excretion of the herbicide 2,4-D occurs readily among dogs after application of the herbicide to lawns. This observation was made particularly during the first 2 days after herbicide application. Hayes et al., (1991) showed a positive association between canine malignant lymphoma, a form of cancer in dogs, and the use of the herbicide 2,4-D by their owners on their lawns and by literature data suggested an increased risk of non-Hodgkin's lymphoma in humans, the histology and epidemiology of which are similar to those of canine malignant lymphoma. Gaines and Kimbrough, (1970) cited by Hansen et al., (1971) reported an increase in mortality among rats whose female parents received approximately 50 mg/kg b. w. per day of 2,4-D in the diet for 3 months before mating and throughout gestation and lactation. Sometimes the influence of toxicants on humans in some cases can be quite disguised or delayed. When hunters use lead pellets, ducks and other species can ingest the lead later, also people or predators that eat these birds can be poisoned (Lightfoot & Yeager, 2008; Ferreyra et al., 2009).

Rodents frequently serve as models to evaluate an exposure risk for humans in ecotoxicological investigations (Shore & Rattner, 2001). Free-living wild rodents are suitable for monitoring the environmental pollution and toxicological risk concerning people living in contaminated regions (O'Brien et al., 1993; Damek-Poprawa & Sawicka-Kapusta, 2003). When small mammals are mentioned, it is generally meant species from two orders: Rodentia and Insectivora. They are used as model organisms, because they have a short life span, co-exist in spatially well-defined small areas, exhibit habitat preferences and feeding behaviour (some are herbivores, omnivores or insectivores) and can be easily caught, marked and studied (Barrett & Pelles, 1999; Metcheva et al., 2003).

Chemical pollutants (which may be considered as component of the general environmental pollution) lead to mutagenesis in somatic and germ cells. As a result of their action the relative frequencies of chromosomal aberrations increase. This fact is used in ecotoxicological investigations to indicate an existing pollution in natural populations (Topashka-Ancheva et al., 2003; Veličković, 2004).

Mutagenic activity of the environmental pollutants is examined on the monitor species considering structural and numerical chromosomal aberrations in somatic cells. In previous investigations some authors (Abramsson-Zetterberg et al., 1997; Ieradi et al., 2003; Zima, 1985) showed that chromosome structures of bone marrow cells in *Apodemus flavicollis* and *Apodemus sylvaticus* are more sensitive to the effect of the environmental pollutants than *Clethrionomys glareolus* and *Microtus arvalis*. Cristaldi et al. (1991) showed an increased micronuclei frequency in bank voles collected in ^{137}Cs contaminated sites. De Souza Bueno et al. (2000) showed a difference in chromosome structure sensitivity of two wild rodent species - *Akodon montensis* and *Oryzomys nigripes* selected as bioindicators in relation to the cytogenetic end points analyzed. These authors pointed out that the mitotic index, the frequency of cells with micronuclei in the bone marrow and peripheral blood, and the frequency of cells with chromosomal aberrations in the bone marrow may reveal a difference in susceptibility to clastogenic agents between the wild species investigated.

Kovalova & Glazko (2006) have revealed the species-specific increase of cytogenetic anomaly frequency in bone marrow cells at a high level of radionuclide pollution and species-specific association between various types of cytogenetic anomalies.

Small mammal species differ in their sensitivity to metal pollution: herbivorous voles and mouse species are regarded as more sensitive than shrew species (Shore & Douben, 1994; Sánchez-Chardi et al. 2007).

Relatively little data is available concerning investigations on changes in chromosomal structure in wild small mammals after an acute treatment of a particular genotoxin under strictly controlled laboratory conditions by comparison with the laboratory mice.

This chapter presents our original findings as well as literature data concerning the effect of some genotoxins on the chromosome structures of four widely distributed in Bulgaria small mammal species and the laboratory ICR mice. These investigations are of present interest, because it is not always correct to extrapolate the genotoxicity findings in laboratory animal models to natural populations. The clastogenic effect of Mitomycin C, $Pb(NO_3)_2$, 2,4-dichlorophenoxyacetic acid (2,4-D) and Tetrahydrofuran was studied on bone marrow cells. The chlorophenoxy herbicide 2,4-D, inorganic lead and organic solvent Tetrahydrofuran are important pollutants of anthropogenic origin. They could affect the chromosomal structures in actively proliferating cell populations, e.g. bone marrow cells and spermatogonial and ovogonial cells as well and thus could be harmful to the genetic material and the organism itself.

1.1 Applied genotoxins

Mutagenic agents we use in this experimental design are one well known clastogen Mitomycin C, as well as some relatively widespread pollutants in the environment - $Pb(NO_3)_2$, 2,4-D and Tetrahydrofuran.

1.1.1 Alkylating agent - mitomycin C (Sigma EC No 200-008-6)

As positive control was selected Mitomycin C - clastogenic agent with proven genotoxic effect, damaging DNA matrix via alkylation. Alkylating compounds are the most active chemical mutagens with high frequency of induced chromosomal aberrations. This compound is a standard laboratory mutagen widely applied on different animal cells (Jena & Bhunya, 1995).

Mitomycin C inhibits DNA synthesis *in vivo* and *in vitro*, reacts covalently with DNA, forming cross-links between the complementary strands of DNA, inhibiting DNA replication (Tomasz et al., 1987), suppress the cell division, thus resulting in induction of chromosomal aberrations.

1.1.2 Lead nitrate $Pb(NO_3)_2$ (Merck, Germany)

Inorganic lead is ubiquitous in the environment because of natural origin or by the industry. Lead is known to replace zinc in many enzymes, including those that are important for proper DNA metabolism and thus can cause fatal injury (Mohammed-Brahim et al., 1985). The lead, cadmium, mercury and arsenic are among the main toxic metals. They accumulate in food chains and have a cumulative effect (Cunningham & Saigo, 1997). Heavy metals often have direct physiologically toxic effects and are sometimes permanently stored or incorporated in living tissues (Bokori et al., 1996).

Lead is a metabolic poison and a neurotoxin that binds to essential enzymes and several other cellular components and inactivates them (Cunningham & Saigo, 1997). Toxic effects of lead are seen on hemopoietic, nervous, gastrointestinal and renal systems (Ma, 1996). Lead can induce single-strand DNA breaks, possibly by competing with metal binding sites in DNA (Shaik et al., 2006).

WHO reported for a few studies in rodents treated with lead salts *in vivo*, which shown small increases in the frequency of chromosomal aberrations and micronuclei in bone-marrow cells, but most of the studies showed no increase (IARC, 1987). Dhir et al., (1993) reported that intraperitoneal (i.p.) injection of low doses lead nitrate in *Mus musculus* caused a significant increase in sister chromatid exchanges rate in bone marrow cells of male Swiss albino mice.

Sharma et al. (1985) found that lead acetate introduced i.p. in ICR mice at doses from 50-200 mg/kg body weight in the 13th day of gestation showed significant increase of sister chromatid exchange rate in maternal bone marrow and foetal liver cells. *In vivo* comet assay studies with Swiss Albino male mice treated by oral intubation with 0.7 up to 89.6 mg/kg body weight $Pb(NO_3)_2$, have shown that lead nitrate causes DNA single strand breaks. No clear dose response between the DNA damage and different doses of $Pb(NO_3)_2$ was detected (Devi et al., 2000).

A significant ecotoxicological risk to a wild population of bank voles (*C. glareolus*), associated with high lead tissue concentration has been estimated by Milton et al. (2003). In Algerian mice (*Mus spretus*), exposed to lead a significant increase in the frequency of micronucleated polychromatic bone marrow erythrocytes and decrease in red blood cells, hematocrit and mean corpuscular hemoglobin were found (Marques et al. 2006).

In a number of studies, lead has been recognized as a potential threat to human health (Goyer, 1993; Jin et al., 2006; Patil et al., 2006). Acidic drinks like tomato juice, fruit juice and others can dissolve lead when packed in inappropriate containers (Karaivanova et al., 2008). This may increase the human risk of lead poisoning. Bilban & Jakopin (2005) found that working in a lead-zinc mine under exposure to radon and heavy metals can result in dramatic consequences for the human DNA (induction of structural chromosomal aberrations) and this is probably more strongly influenced by heavy metals than by radon.

At toxic concentrations, lead acetate and lead nitrate can inhibit DNA repair and damage DNA acting as a comutagen and possibly a cocarcinogen (Roy & Rossman, 1992).

1.1.3 2,4-dichlorophenoxyacetic acid (2,4-D) (Merck, Germany)

2,4-D is an alkylchlorophenoxy herbicide and one of the most frequently used herbicides worldwide as growth regulator for a variety of broad-leaf weeds (while sparing grasses) in agricultural, forestry, and aquatic sites. This herbicide is synthetic structural analogue of natural auxin indole-3-il-acetic acid, which plays a crucial role in division, differentiation and elongation of plant cells. Overdose application of synthetic auxins induces disorganized growth and death in susceptible plant species. There are contradictory results in the literature about the toxicity and possible mutagenic effect of the herbicide 2,4-D, but some investigations emphasize on the observed cellular mutations after exposure which can lead to cancer, immunosuppression, reproductive damage and neurotoxicity (Hayes et al., 1991; Amer & Aly, 2001; Charles et al., 1996b; Rosso et al., 2000). Charles et al., (1996a) found no oncogenic effect of 0-300 mg/kg 2,4-D in mice or 0-150 mg/kg in rats, although slightly increase in primary hepatocellular adenomas were observed in female mice, but with lack of dose response. *In vivo* studies found that 2,4-D included chromatid breaks, chromatid fragments, ring chromosomes, dicentric chromosomes, and chromosome fragments in bone marrow cells in rats (Adhikari & Grover, 1988) and increased rates of sister chromatid exchanges were determined in cultured human lymphocytes (Turkula & Jalal, 1985) if applied at lower dosage. Gonzalez et al. (2005) found that doses of 6 ppm and 10 ppm 2,4-D increased sister chromatid exchanges, reduced mitotic index and increased DNA damage in Chinese hamster ovary cells. In studies in mice Charles et al. (1999) indicated that 2,4-D clearly demonstrates a lack of cytogenetic damage at any dose level in the bone marrow micronucleus test. These authors also concluded that 2,4-D is not genotoxic in mammalian systems *in vivo*. Holland et al. (2002) found no statistically significant increase in MN frequency after exposure of 2,4-D in human peripheral blood lymphocytes. Injection of about 2.0 mg 2,4-D into fertile 60 g hen eggs was found to be embryotoxic and decreased in some cases the viability of the chicks, while immersion in a five percent solution had only a moderate effect on hatching (Gyrd-Hansen & Dalgaard-Mikkelsen, 1974). Arias (2003) reported a positive linear correlation between the increase of sister chromatid exchanges and doses (0.5, 1, 2 and 4 mg/embryo) in chicken eggs treated with commercial 2,4-D. Despite these contradictory results, reviews of 2,4-D (Sierra Club of Canada, 2005; Bukowska, 2006; NRDC, 2008; Water Hyacinth Control Program, 2009) determined this herbicide as a genotoxic agent.

1.1.4 Tetrahydrofuran (THF) (Merck, Germany)

THF is a synthesized organic compound, which cannot be found in the natural environment (ACGIH, 2001). THF is used as a solvent in the manufacture of adhesives, lacquers, printing inks, fats, oils, unvulcanized rubber, etc. Its active ingredient furan is released by combustion of organic waste and thermal treatment of food. Furan is toxic and is a proven carcinogen in laboratory animals (Heppner & Schlatter, 2007).

The probable oral lethal dose of THF in humans is 50-500 mg/kg (Gosselin, 1976). Katahira et al. (1982) evaluated LD_{50} as 1900 mg/kg in rats and 2500 mg/kg in mice after acute toxicity of 20% THF in olive oil by i.p. injection. Chhabra et al. (1998) found a clear evidence of carcinogenic activity in female $B6C3F_1$ mice observing increased incidences of hepatocellular neoplasms at the 1800 ppm exposure level, but these authors did not observe carcinogenic effect of THF in female rats and male mice. Inhalation studies with rats and $B6C3F_1$ mice also provided evidence of carcinogenic activity for THF (Gamer et al., 2002).

THF was not mutagenic in *Salmonella*, micronucleus and DEL tests and did not induce sister chromatid exchanges or chromosomal aberrations in ovary cells (Gamer et al., 2002). According to the data of NTP (1998) in male $B6C3F_1$ mice after i.p. injection of THF at doses of up to 2000 mg/kg significant increase in the number of chromosomal aberrations in the bone marrow cells was not observed. Despite that, ACGIH (2010) confirmed that THF is animal carcinogen with unknown relevance to humans.

1.2 Experimental animals

Model species have been selected to meet the following conditions: they are widespread and are situated low in the food chain, have short reproductive cycle and left several generations a year. Mice of the genus *Apodemus* and voles are well-accepted zoomonitors in environmental pollution studies (Metcheva et al., 1996, 2001). They possess well-studied karyotypes with relatively low number of chromosomes and clearly distinguishable chromosomal morphology (Belcheva et al., 1987; Zima, 2004).

The laboratory mice are well known experimental animals, frequently used as controls in laboratory research. They are the most commonly used mammalian model, more common than rats (Gerasimova & Topashka-Ancheva, 2010).

In this investigation, five small mammal species were used:

Apodemus sp. (Kaup, 1829) The description of the karyotype of *Apodemus sp.* was made by R. Matthey in 1936, based on material from Eastern Europe (2n=48, NF=48) and later by other authors (Belcheva et al., 1987; Zima & Kral, 1984). X-chromosome is the largest and Y is the smallest it the karyotype. All authosomes are acrocentric.

Clethrionomys glareolus (Schreber, 1780) (2n=56, NF=59) karyotype consists of 26 pairs of acrocentric and one pair of small metacentric autosomes. X-chromosome is large acrocentric, one of the largest in the complement, while Y is small metacentric like the materials from Central Europe (Belcheva et al., 1987).

Microtus (s.str.) *arvalis* (Pallas, 1778) (2n=46, In Bulgaria NFa=80, NF=84) karyotype is identical with the form "*arvalis*", known from Western and Central Europe; most of the chromosome pairs are metacentric (Belcheva et al., 1977).

Mus spicilegus (Petényi, 1882) karyotype is described for the first time by Painter in 1928 (2n=40). All 19 authosome pairs are acrocentric. Y chromosome is very small and an X chromosome is among the largest acrocentrics of the complement (Mitsainas et al., 2009).

This morphology is characteristic for all subspecies of *Mus musculus musculus* (*domesticus*, *musculus*, *castaneus*, and *bactrianus*) as well as the laboratory lines and the closely related species *Mus spretus* and *Mus macedonicus*.

Mus spicilegus was selected, as it is one of the most frequent species in agroecosystems along with voles.

Male and female laboratory white mice ICR (2n=40) (♂♀=53), weighting 20±1,5 g were delivered from the Slivnitza animal breeding house of the Bulgarian Academy of Sciences, Sofia. Animals were kept at standard conditions at temperature 20-22°C, photoperiod 7am to 7pm, free access to standard animal food for laboratory animals - "Rodents" (produced by Vitaprot-Ltd., Kostinbrod, Bulgaria, according prescription 456-1-12) and water.

All small mammal species originated from several conditionally unpolluted regions in Bulgaria: Rila Natural Park, Vitosha Nature Park, Kresna Gorge and the vicinities of Pleven region. *Apodemus* sp. (♂♀=80), *Clethrionomys glareolus* (♂♀=44), *Microtus arvalis* (♂♀=61), *Mus spicilegus* (♂♀=71).

The experimental treatment of the wild model species was conducted not earlier than 48 hours after capture and the structural changes in the chromosomes were scored 24 hours after treatment with the genotoxins.

The experiments were conducted according to approved protocols, and in compliance with the requirements of the European Convention for Protection of Vertebrate Animals used for experimental and other Specific Purposes and the current Bulgarian laws and regulations.

2. Cytogenetical analysis

Bone marrow is one of the most convenient tissues for testing the mutagenic effects of environmental factors due to the low frequency of spontaneous chromosomal aberrations, high cell proliferative activity, relatively rapid and simple method of making the preparations. The prevailing forms of chromosomal damage are those of the chromatid type. The cytogenetical method applied is intended to show the sensitivity of chromosomal aberration assay in animal's bone marrow to determine whether certain components of the environment can induce chromosomal aberrations with a frequency that is significantly higher compared with their frequency in the control animals or in animals from unaffected areas.

Mitomycin C (3.5 mg/kg b.w.) (Sigma EC No 200-008-6), Pb(NO3)2 (200 mg/kg b.w.) (Merck, Germany), 2,4-D (3.5 mg/kg b.w.) (Merck, Germany) and THF (3.8 mg/kg b.w.) (Merck, Germany) were injected intraperitoneally (i.p.) only once. Control animals received only 0.9% NaCl solution. All the genotoxins applied were dissolved in 0.9% NaCl solution. The accurate number of males and females used in the experiments for each toxicant applied is presented in relevant tables.

Our previous data (Venkov et al., 2000) on low clastogenic and multiple effect of 2,4-D which is widely used in the treatment of weeds in agroecosystems gave us reasons to expand our experiments. The herbicide 2,4-D (3.5 mg/kg b.w.) was introduced i.p. three consecutive times at intervals of 48 hours (total 96 hours). Bone marrow cell samples for cytogenetical analysis were prepared 24 hours after the third and last injection of the herbicide (total 120 hours after the initial herbicide treatment).

The cytogenetical analysis was mainly performed according to the protocol described by Preston et al. (1987). To accumulate a sufficient number of metaphases in order to obtain metaphase chromosomes suitable for cytogenetic analysis, one hour before bone marrow cell isolation a mitotic inhibitor colchicine – 0.04 mg /g b.w. was injected. Animals were euthanized by diethyl ether, bone marrow cells were flushed from femur and hypotonized in a 0.075 M potassium chloride at 37°C for 15 min. Thereafter the cells were fixed in cold methanol: glacial acetic acid (3:1), resuspended and dropped on precleaned cold wet slides and air dried. The slides were stained in 5 % Giemsa solution (Sigma Diagnostic). Up to 50 well-scattered metaphase plates were analyzed from each animal using light microscopy (Cetopan Reichert, Austria) x 1000.

The main types of aberrations – breaks, fragments, exchanges (centromer/centromeric fusions, telomere/telomeric fusions) and pericentric inversions were separately scored.

2.1 Statistical analysis

The frequencies of chromosomal aberrations were determined for each animal. The mean ±SD for each group was calculated and the data was statistically evaluated for their significance by analysis of variance using the Student t test. Statistical significance is expressed as $p<0.001$; $p<0.01$; $p<0.05$; $p>0.05$ - (not significant).

3. Results and discussion

The chromosome aberration frequencies in the analyzed bone marrow cells of all five small mammal species investigated are presented in Tables 1-4. The values of the metaphases with aberrations in ICR mice control group are 1.0±0.3%, 3.25±0.36% in *M. spicilegus*, 3.43±0.57% in *M. arvalis*, 1.2±0.42% in *C. glareolus* and 2.66±0.4% in *Apodemus sp*. These percentages of aberrant metaphases were in most cases within the range of frequencies, determined in cells of various small mammal species captured in different wild habitats (Topashka et al., 2003).

There was no statistically significant difference in the percentage of chromosomal aberrations for each experimental group between males and females after experimental treatment with all toxicants under present investigation. That allowed combining the results for both sexes and presenting them as mean ± SD%.

3.1 Mitomycin C clastogenicity

The chosen dose of Mitomycin C was administrated i.p. in all experimental animals and the percentages of chromosomal aberrations are presented in Table 1.

In all investigated species the experimental treated groups showed reliably higher percentage of damaged cells in comparison with the untreated controls ($p<0.01$).

The highest percentage of cells with chromosomal aberrations was observed within the treated group of the laboratory mice ICR (38.42±1.88%) followed by its relative species *M. spicilegus* (21.6±1.45%). Significant reduction of the amount of cells with aberrations in bone marrow of the treated *Apodemus sp.* was observed (11.01±0.81%). The lowest values of cells with aberrations appeared in the species of family Cricetidae: *C. glareolus* (10.38±1.57%) and *M. arvalis* (10.72±0.28%). Obviously, ICR mice showed a three-fold higher sensitivity in comparison with the treated *C. glareolus*, *M. arvalis* and *Apodemus sp.* ($p<0.001$).

These results indicate that all wild small mammal species injected i.p. with Mitomycin C showed significantly lower karyotype sensitivity in comparison with the ICR mice (p≤0.01). The chromosome structure of both treated species of genus *Mus* is more susceptible to the action of the alkylating agent Mitomycin C (p<0.05).

Chromatid breaks and fragments as though chromosomal rearrangements (centromeric fusions (c/c), telomeric fusions (t/t), pericentric inversions and taranslocations) were separately scored. Breaks and fragments significantly prevail over the chromosomal type aberrations (from 74% of all aberrations observed in laboratory mice, 75% in *Apodemus sp.*, 83.3% in *C. glareolus*, 91.7% in *M. spicilegus* up to 96% in *M. arvalis*). The share of breaks and fragments appears to be the highest in *M. spicilegus, M. arvalis* and *C. glareolus* and lowest in ICR mice.

Compound		Time after treatment	Number of metaphases scored	Type of chromosomal aberrations					Pericentric inversions	Polyploid cells	Percentage of cells with aberrations (X±m)
				Breaks	Fragments	Rearrangements					
						c/c	t/t	c/t			
ICR	Mit. C	24 h	6♂4♀ 500	66	82	38	8	0	6	0	38.42 ± 1.88
ICR	control	24h	5♂1♀ 250	3	0	2	0	0	0	0	1.00 ± 0.33
M. spicilegus	Mit. C	24 h	6♂4♀ 500	49	50	5	2	0	2	0	21.6 ± 1.45
M. spicilegus	control	24h	5♂3♀ 400	7	4	0	0	0	0	0	3.25 ± 0.36
M. arvalis	Mit. C	24 h	10♂9♀ 902	64	32	0	0	0	4	0	10.72 ± 0.28
M. arvalis	control	24h	7♂ 350	8	4	0	0	0	0	0	3.43 ± 0.57
C. glareolus	Mit. C	24 h	2♂2♀ 165	9	6	1	1	0	1	0	10.38 ± 1.57
C. glareolus	control	24h	5♂5♀ 471	3	2	1	0	0	0	4	1.20 ± 0.42
Apodemus sp.	Mit. C	24 h	10♂8♀ 911	33	45	10	4	0	12	34	11.01 ± 0.81
Apodemus sp.	control	24h	5♂6♀ 498	9	4	0	0	0	0	0	2.66 ± 0.40

Table 1. Number and frequency of chromosomal aberrations found in ICR strain laboratory mice, *M. spicilegus, M. arvalis, C. glareolus* and *Apodemus sp.* after experimental treatment with Mitomycin C (3.5mg/kg b.w./24 h).

The prevalence of breaks and fragments in the treated groups of all five species is a result of specific action of alkylating agent Mitomycin C.

Jena and Bhunya (1995) showed that Mitomycin C applied on bone marrow cells of *Gallus domesticus* provoked chromatid and isochromatid breaks, deletions and exchanges. The mechanism of action of Mitomycin C at the molecular level is due to the formation of DNA-DNA crosslinking adducts (Tomasz et al., 1987). The prevalence of breaks and fragments observed is a result of the biological action of Mitomycin C, and the number of the affected metaphases depends on the karyotype stability of the studied model species.

We found that the centromeric/centromeric fusions (c/c fusions) are more frequent in ICR mice than in all other species investigated. The rate of exchanges between non-homologous chromosomes in the mouse is particularly high. This is facilitated by the acrocentric nature of mouse's chromosomes. The acrocentric chromosomes in genus *Mus* are prone to c/c fusions because of the specific structure of the centromeric regions. This phenomenon is due to single strand's breaks in the minor SAT DNA located in the centromeric regions of mice chromosomes (Kipling et al., 1994).

In the Mitomycin C treated groups pericentric inversions – 1.33±0.36% for *Apodemus sp.* group and 1.2±0.5% for ICR mice and 3.77±0.78% polyploid metaphases (4n, 8n) in *Apodemus sp.* were also observed. In the polyploid cells some of the chromosomes were also damaged (fragments and pericentric inversions were seen).

3.2 Pb (NO₃)₂ clastogenicity

A total number of 49 animals from all five rodent species were treated with lead nitrate (200 mg/kg b.w.). More than 2370 metaphase plates were analized. The results are presented in Table 2.

The highest percentage of metaphases with aberrations was scored in slides of bone marrow cell population in ICR mice (11.03±0.89%). Close to these values are calculated in slides of *M. spicilegus* (9.6±0.4%). In both vole species (*M. arvalis* and *C. glareolus*) a tendency to reduce the yield of chromosomal aberrations is observed - respectively 8.93±0.61% and 8.8±0.53%. Despite the differences in absolute values of this index reported for *M. arvalis* and *C. glareolus* and laboratory mice these differences are with low level of confidence ($p \leq 0.05$).

Compound		Time after treat ment	Number of metaphase s scored	Breaks	Fragments	c/c	t/t	c/c	Pericentric inversions	Polyploid cells	Percentage of cells with aberrations (X±m)
							Rearrangements				
ICR	Pb(NO₃)₂	24h	6♂5♀ 550	30	11	18	2	0	0	0	11.03 ± 0.89
ICR	control	24h	5♂1♀ 250	3	0	2	0	0	0	0	1.00 ± 0.33
M. spicilegus	Pb(NO₃)₂	24h	5♂5♀ 500	22	14	11	1	0	0	1	9.60 ± 0.40
M. spicilegus	control	24h	5♂3♀ 400	7	4	0	0	0	0	0	3.25 ± 0.36
M. arvalis	Pb(NO₃)₂	24h	4♂3♀ 307	20	5	0	2	0	0	0	8.93 ± 0.61
M. arvalis	control	24h	7♂ 350	8	4	0	0	0	0	0	3.43 ± 0.57
C. glareolus	Pb(NO₃)₂	24h	7♂3♀ 500	16	16	8	3	0	0	30	8.80 ± 0.53
C. glareolus	control	24h	5♂5♀ 471	3	2	1	0	0	0	4	1.20 ± 0.42
Apodemus sp.	Pb(NO₃)₂	24h	7♂4♀ 520	20	4	0	0	0	9	12	6.00 ± 0.60
Apodemus sp.	control	24h	5♂6♀ 498	9	4	0	0	0	0	0	2.66 ± 0.40

Table 2. Number and frequency of chromosomal aberrations found in ICR strain laboratory mice, *M. spicilegus*, *M. arvalis*, *C. glareolus* and *Apodemus sp.* after experimental treatment with Pb(NO₃)₂ (200mg/kg b.w./24 h)

The lowest percentage of metaphases with damaged chromosomes is evaluated in the group of *Apodemus sp.* (6.0±0.60%). These values are significantly lower than the percentages of cells with aberrations calculated for the other four small mammal species ($p<0.01$ to $p<0.001$).

Based on the experimental data the laboratory ICR mice and *M. spicilegus* showed a tendency of greater sensitivity to the damaging effect of Pb(NO₃)₂ in comparison with the other three wild species investigated. The high percentage of aberrant metaphases detected in treated *M. spicilegus* experimental group correlated with the data obtained by Topashka-Ancheva and Metcheva (1999) for *M. macedonicus* samples (8.89±2.34% for males and 10.46±0.93% for females) collected near the heavy metal polluted region of lead-zinc factory in the vicinities of Asenovgrad (Bulgaria).

The study showed that *Apodemus sp.* has significantly greater stability of the karyotype in comparison with ICR mice, *M. spicilegus*, *M. arvalis* and *C. glareolus* exposed to lead nitrate. This is an important conclusion in the use of *Apodemus sp.* in the ecotoxicological studies concerning the damaging influence of lead as environmental pollutant.

Chromosomal rearrangements of chromatid type - breaks and fragments predominated in all samples analyzed (from 61.1% in ICR mice up to 92% in *M. arvalis*).

The rise of chromatid type breaks and exchanges is mainly a result of double strand breaks generated in postreplicative DNA in later S phase and in G_2 phase (Hagmar et al., 2004). Chromatid type aberrations (breaks and fragments) may arise also in response to single strand breaks induced in early S phase. Chromatid breaks observed in metaphases would result from incomplete or failed repair (Pfeiffer et al., 2000). Chromatid type aberrations are usually generated by S-phase-dependent clastogens (e.g. chemical agents) (Mateuca et al., 2006). Single strand breaks resulting from lead influence were reported by Valverde et al. (2002), and Shaik et al. (2006).

The data of our experiments for the high presence of chromatid breaks in the examined small mammal species, compared with the data of other authors, provide evidence that lead is mainly S-phase-dependent clastogen. Jagetia and Aruna (1998) reported that lead induced micronuclei were observed even at very low doses. After i.p. treatment with lead nitrate, the highest increases in the frequencies of micronucleated polychromatic erythrocytes were observed after treatment with 80 mg/kg b.w. in mouse bone marrow at 12, 24 and 36 h post-treatment. These authors suggested that the increase of micronuclei might be due to the induction of DNA strand breaks by lead nitrate.

In the ICR, *M. spicilegus* and *C. glareolus* groups treated with $Pb(NO_3)_2$ metaphases with centromeric fusions were also observed (28%, 23%and 20% respectively). Centromeric/centromeric fusions were practically not detected in *Apodemus sp.* and *M. arvalis* treated with $Pb(NO_3)_2$.

The results obtained in this study are in agreement with those of Nayak et al. (1989) who reported that lead nitrate (100-200 mg/kg b.w.) on gestational day 9 exhibited a moderate, but significantly increased sister chromatid exchanges in maternal bone marrow of ICR Swiss Webster mice. Several specific chromosomal aberrations, mostly deletions in maternal bone marrow and fetal cells were also calculated.

3.3 2,4-dichlorophenoxyacetic acid (2,4-D) clastogenicity

The quantitative data from the metaphase analysis of the bone marrow cells are summarized on Table 3.

The cytogenetic analysis carried out upon well spread metaphase plates evidenced that single administration of 2,4-D induced aberrations such as breaks, fragments and exchanges. Seldom were observed more than one aberration per analyzed metaphase. In proliferating bone marrow cell populations of all small mammal species investigated the percentages of chromosomal aberrations were approximately equal - from 4.55±0.39% in *M. spicilegus* to 5.8±0.55% in *C. glareolus*.

After triple introduction of 3.5 mg/kg b.w. 2,4-D, the damaged cells of the treated animals were at reliably higher percentages. The highest, but almost equal percentages of chromosomal aberrations were evaluated in ICR mice (11.5±0.5%) and *Apodemus sp.* (10.33±1.08). The values were significantly higher compared to those obtained after single i.p. injection of 2,4-D (p<0.001). In *M. spicilegus* and *M. arvalis* experimental groups these values were lower (7.1±0.67% and 6.16±0.60%, respectively), but they were significantly higher than the data obtained after single dose only.

The types of chromosomal aberrations in samples after single and triple treatment were quite similar (breaks, fragments and centromeric/centromeric fusions, and occasionally telomeric/telomeric fusions). The telomeric/telomeric fusions are a result of terminal deletions and fusion in the region of so-called sticky edges. The higher number of metaphases with centromeric/centromeric chromosomal fusions in ICR mice and *M. spicilegus* can be explained again with the peculiarities of their acrocentric karyotype. Centromeric/centromeric fusions in the samples of *M. spicilegus* reached 60.5% after triple herbicide treatment.

Compound		Time after treatment	Number of metaphases scored	Type of chromosomal aberrations					Pericentric inversions	Polyploid cells	Percentage of cells with aberrations (X±m)
				Breaks	Fragments	Rearrangements					
						c/c	t/t	c/t			
ICR	2,4-D	24 h	5♂5♀ 500	8	6	9	0	0	0	0	4,6 ± 0,43
ICR	2,4-D triple	24 h	8♂ 400	14	16	16	0	0	0	0	11,5 ± 0,5
ICR	control	24h	5♂1♀ 250	3	0	2	0	0	0	0	1,0 ± 0,33
M. spicilegus	2,4-D	24 h	4♂7♀ 550	12	6	6	1	1	0	1	4,55 ± 0,39
M. spicilegus	2,4-D triple	24 h	5♂5♀ 550	10	5	23	1	0	0	0	7,1 ± 0,67
M. spicilegus	2,4-D control	24 h	8♂2♀ 500	3	10	5	0	0	0	1	3,67 ± 0,61
M. arvalis	2,4-D	24 h	5♂5♀ 491	19	2	2	0	0	0	2	4,72 ± 0,48
M. arvalis	2,4-D triple	24 h	3♂6♀ 430	13	10	0	0	0	0	1	6,16 ± 0,60
M. arvalis	control	24h	7♂ 350	8	4	0	0	0	0	0	3.43 ± 0.57
C. glareolus	2,4-D	24 h	4♂6♀ 500	19	7	2	1	0	0	2	5,8 ± 0,55
C. glareolus	control	24h	5♂5♀ 471	3	2	1	0	0	0	4	1,2 ± 0,42
Apodemus sp.	2,4-D	24 h	6♂6♀ 612	15	11	4	1	0	0	4	5,0 ± 0,52
Apodemus sp.	2,4-D triple	24 h	4♂2♀ 300	7	24	0	0	0	0	13	10,33 ± ,08
Apodemus sp.	2,4-D control	24 h	6♀ 300	4	4	1	0	0	0	1	3,0 ± 0,45

Table 3. Number and frequency of chromosomal aberrations found in ICR strain laboratory mice, *M. spicilegus, M. arvalis, C. glareolus* and *Apodemus sp.* after experimental treatment with 2,4-dichlorophenoxyacetic acid 2,4-D (3,5 mg/kg b.w.)

Calculated as percentage of the total number of damaged cells, the amount of the chromatid type aberrations (breaks and fragments) ranged from 60% in ICR mice up to 100% in *M. arvalis* and *Apodemus sp.* after triple treatment with 2,4-D.

We found that 2,4-dichlorophenoxyacetic acid exhibits moderate damaging effect on the chromosomes of the studied small mammal species. This damaging effect is increased because of the triple herbicide introduction. These results are in agreement with the data of Amer and Aly (2001), who found a significant increase in the percentage of chromosomal aberrations in bone marrow and spermatocyte cells after oral administration of 3.3 mg/kg b.w. 2,4-D for three and five consecutively introduced applications of the herbicide. At the same time, a single dose of 1.7 mg/kg and 3.3 mg/kg b.w. did not show a significant increase of the chromosomal aberrations in bone marrow and spermatocyte cells of the male Swiss mice. These authors found that 2,4-D induce structural and numerical chromosomal aberrations in bone marrow cells and a dose-dependent relationship in the percentage of metaphases with chromosomal aberrations (6.8±0.73% 24 hours after single oral treatment with 3.3 mg/kg b.w.). Our results were quite similar – 4.6±0.43% after single i.p injection in ICR mice and 11.5±0.5% after triple introduction of the herbicide.

In earlier studies Venkov et al. (2000) in C57/Bl mice treated i.p. with 3.5 mg/kg 2,4-D found that this herbicide exhibits a positive reply for chromosomal aberrations and significantly reduced mitotic activity with *in vivo* test. These authors found that 2,4-D induced 5.50±1.90% chromosomal aberrations 24 hours after i.p. treatment with significant prevalence of centromeric fusions, but also observed that 2,4-D had weaker clastogenic effect compared to the positive control Mitomycin C (23.35±0.95%). From the results of their experiment, it can be suggested that the genetic damage caused by phenoxy herbicide should not be ignored. We confirmed and enlarged their results in our experimental design that in all five small mammal species investigated the equal dose of 3.5mg/kg 2,4-D possessed significantly lower clastogenic effect compared to the same dose of the alkylating agent Mitomycin C. Our results obtained in *in vivo* investigations support the results of Gandhi et al. (2003), that a potential genetic hazard exists because of the widespread use of 2,4-D in agroecosystems. Since the genetic damage may result from the exposure to agricultural chemicals in the environment, there is a further need to evaluate the potential hazard that 2,4-D may exhibit to animal species living in the wild.

3.4 THF clastogenicity

The data of the cytogenetic analysis conducted on the treated bone marrow cells with 3.8 mg/kg THF on small mammal species is presented on Table 4.

Compound		Time after treatment	Number of metaphases scored	Breaks	Fragments	Rearrangements c/c	Rearrangements t/t	Rearrangements c/t	Pericentric inversions	Polyploid cells	Percentage of cells with aberrations (X±m)
ICR	THF	24h	4♂4♀ 400	19	15	23	2	0	0	0	14.75±0.92
ICR	control	24h	5♂1♀ 250	3	0	2	0	0	0	0	1.00 ± 0.33
M. spicilegus	THF	24h	4♂8♀ 600	20	19	6	0	0	0	0	7.50 ± 0.44
M. spicilegus	control	24h	5♂3♀ 400	7	4	0	0	0	0	0	3.25 ± 0.36
M. arvalis	THF	24h	4♂5♀ 384	20	5	0	1	0	0	2	6.93 ± 0.52
M. arvalis	control	24h	7♂ 350	8	4	0	0	0	0	0	3.43 ± 0.57
C. glareolus	THF	24h	4♂6♀ 500	19	12	3	3	0	0	2	7.40 ± 0.43
C.glareolus	control	24h	5♂5♀ 471	3	2	1	0	0	0	4	1.20 ± 0.42
Apodemus sp.	THF	24h	11♂3♀ 621	19	23	2	0	0	0	7	6.85 ± 0.41
Apodemus sp.	control	24h	5♂6♀ 498	9	4	0	0	0	0	0	2.66 ± 0.40

Table 4. Number and frequency of chromosomal aberrations found in ICR strain laboratory mice, *M. spicilegus*, *M. arvalis*, *C. glareolus* and *Apodemus sp.* after experimental treatment with THF (3.8mg/kg b.w./24 h).

The results showed that the highest percentage of cells with aberrant chromosomes was evaluated in ICR mice (14.75±0.92%). Bone marrow cells of four other species studied possessed great similarity in their reaction to the genotoxin applied. The data about the absolute values for the percentage of cells with aberrations in *M. spicilegus*, *M. arvalis*, *C. glareolus* and *Apodemus sp.* did not significantly differ (p>0.05). In all samples analyzed chromatid-type aberrations (breaks and fragments) were predominating. The highest percentages of breaks and fragments among all aberrations scored were observed in *M. arvalis* (96%) and *Apodemus sp.* (95%), and the lowest in the ICR mice group (57.6%). In the ICR group high percentage of cells with chromosomal exchanges were scored (42.4% aberrant cells with c/c and t/t fusions).

It should be noted however that values for chromosomal aberration obtained after treatment with THF were significantly lower than those with Mitomycin C. These findings suggest a moderate clastogenic effect of the studied genotoxin. There was no statistical significance in the values of aberrant metaphases obtained in experimental groups treated with THF and $Pb(NO_3)_2$ (p>0.05). ICR mice, *M. spicilegus* and *M. arvalis* showed higher chromosome sensitivity to the THF effect compared to the herbicide 2,4-D (p<0.001; p<0.01, respectively). Such dependency was not observed in the aberrant metaphases in *C. glareolus* and *Apodemus sp.* after single i.p. treatement with 2,4-D.

The results obtained in our cytogenetic study evidence that THF have a clastogenic effect and confirm previous data (Gamer et al., 2002) showing an increase of sister chromatid exchanges and chromosomal aberrations following an i.p. treatment with that genotoxin.

4. Conclusion

The effect of various genotoxins on the chromosome set has been intensively studied. Studies on the structural changes in the karyotypes of small mammal species are of a great interest. In this context we investigated the effect of certain genotoxins (Mitomycin C, Lead nitrate, herbicide 2,4-D and THF) on the chromosome integrity of ICR laboratory mice, *M. spicilegus*, *M. arvalis*, *C. glareolus* and *Apodemus sp.* in experimental conditions. Original data about the amount and the type of chromosome aberrations were obtained.

All four wild small mammal species (*M. spicilegus*, *M. arvalis*, *C. glareolus* and *Apodemus sp.*) and the ICR laboratory mice used in this experimental design have responded by changes in chromosomal structure after the intraperitoneal injection of all genotoxins applied.

All the injected compounds caused predominantly chromatid breaks and fragments in small mammal species investigated. Chromosomal exchanges (c/c and t/t fusions) were characteristic mainly for ICR mice and *M. spicilegus* because of their acrocentric type of chromosomes.

The highest karyotype sensitivity to the genotoxins applied was detected in the ICR mouse karyotype, followed by its closely related species *M. spicilegus*.

Both vole species *M. arvalis* and *C. glareolus* showed a similar chromosomal fragility towards the action of most genotoxins applied (Mitomycin C, $Pb(NO_3)_2$ and THF). The karyotype of *Apodemus sp.* showed relatively highest chromosomal stability to the genotoxic action of lead nitrate and Mitomycin C. The percentages of metaphases with aberrant chromosomes in

Apodemus sp. groups after treatment with the herbicide 2,4-D and THF were similar to those of *M. spicilegus*, *M. arvalis* and *C. glareolus*.

The highly pronounced karyotype reaction of *M. spicilegus* to the genotoxins applied and its attachment to agroecosystems would allow the use of this species in genetical monitoring. *M. spicilegus* also has an advantage because of its relatively small chromosomal set (2n=40) and acrocentric type of chromosomes, which allows fast and accurate evaluation of the arising structural chromosomal aberrations. As we found that the chromosome fragility of both *Mus* species (laboratory ICR mice and *M. spicilegus*) was rather similar, the laboratory mouse may also be used successfully in a relatively accurate assessment concerning the genotoxic effects of various xenobiotics introduced in one way or another in agroecosystems.

In so far as the three species – *M. arvalis*, *C. glareolus* and *Apodemus sp.* also react with changes in the structure of their chromosomes under influence of various genotoxins, each of them can be used for the needs of the impact as well as the background genetic monitoring.

Finally, chromosome set of the studied model species possess different sensitivity to the effect of the genotoxin applied.

In all small mammal species investigated the type of chromosomal aberrations observed depends on the chemical nature of the mutagen applied, while the amount of the damaged cells is determined by the karyotype stability.

The specific sensitivity of the chromosomes observed in all used wild small mammal species imposed as zoomonitors is a very important characteristic that must be borne in mind when these species are used for environmental genetic risk assessment.

5. Acknowledgements

This study is supported by project "Development of scientific potential in terms of faunistic diversity and environmental protection", funded by Ministry of Education, Youth and Science, Republic of Bulgaria, BG051PO001.3.3-04/41 and Institute of biodiversity and ecosystem research, Bulgarian Academy of Sciences, Sofia, Bulgaria.

6. References

Abramsson-Zetterberg, L.; Grawe, J. & Zetterber,g G. (1997). Spontaneous and radiation-induced micronuclei in erythrocytes from four species of wild rodents: A comparison with CBA mice. *Mutat Res.*, Vol.393, No.1-2, (September 1997), pp. 55–71, ISSN 0027-5107

ACGIH (American Conference of Governmental Industrial Hygienists). (2001) Tetrahydrofuran. In: Documentation of the threshold limit values and biological exposure indices. Cincinnati, OH: American Conference of Governmental Industrial Hygienists.

ACGIH. (2010). *Threshold Limit Values for Chemical Substances and Physical Agents and Biological Exposure Indices.* American Conference of Governmental Industrial Hygienists TLVs and BEIs. Cincinnati, OH 2010, p. 56.

Adhikari, N. & Grover, I.S. (1988). Genotoxic effects of some systemic pesticides: *In vivo* chromosomal aberrations in bone marrow cells in rats. *Environ. Molec. Mutagen.*, Vol.12, No.2, (January 1988), pp. 235-242, ISSN 0893-6692

Albertini, R.J.; Anderson, D., Douglas, G.R., Hagmar, L., Hemmimki, K., Merlo, F., Natarajan, A.T., Norppa, H., Shuker, D.E., Tice, R., Waters, M.D. & Aitio, A. (2000). IPCS guidelines for the monitoring of genotoxic effects of carcinogens in humans. International Programme on Chemical Safety. *Mutation Res.*, Vol.463, No.2, (August 2000), pp. 111-172, ISSN 1383-5742

Amer, S.M. & Aly, F.A.E. (2001). Genotoxic effect of 2,4-dichlorophenoxy acetic acid and its metabolite 2,4-dichlorophenol in mouse. *Mutation Research*, Vol.494, No.1, (July 2001), pp. 1–12, ISSN 1383-5718

Arias, E. (2003). Sister chromatid exchange induction by the herbicide 2,4-dichlorophenoxyacetic acid in chick embryos. *Ecotoxicology and Environmental Safety*, Vol.55, No.3, (July 2003), pp. 338-343, ISSN 0147-6513

Barrett, G.W. & Pelles, J.D. (1999). Small mammal ecology: A landscape perspective. In: *Landscape Ecology of Small mammals*, Barrett, G. W. & Peles. J. D (Eds.), pp. 347, Springer, ISBN 978-0387986463, New York

Belcheva, R.; Peshev, Ts. & Radjably, S. (1977). Analysis of chromosomal number of Bulgarian common vole (Microtus arvalis). *Zool jurn.*, Vol. 56, No2, pp. 315-317 (In Russian).

Belcheva, R.; Topashka-Ancheva, M., Pechev, Ts. & Gerasimov, S. (1987). Karyological investigations on some rodent species in Bulgaria. In: *Achievements of modern Bulgarian Zoology*, Sofia, BAS, pp. 376-379.

Bender, M.A.; Awa, A.A., Brooks, A.L., Evans, H.J., Groer, P.G., Littlefield, L.G., Pereira, C., Preston, R.J. & Wachholz, B.W. (1988). Current status of cytogenetic procedures to detect and quantify previous exposures to radiation. *Mutat. Res.*, Vol.196, No.2, (September 1988), pp. 103–159, ISSN 0027-5107

Bilban, M. & Jakopin, C.B. (2005) Incidence of cytogenetic damage in lead-zinc mine workers exposed to radon. *Mutagenesis,* Vol. 20, No.3, (May 2005), pp. 187-191, ISSN 02678357

Bokori, J.; Fekete, S., Glavits, R., Kadar, I., Konez, J. & Kovari, L. (1996). Complex study of the physiological role of cadmium IV. Effects of prolonged dietary exposure of broiler chickens to lead. *Acta vet. Hung.*, Vol.44, pp. 57–74, ISSN 0236-6290

Bukowska, B. (2006).Toxicity of 2,4-Dichlorophenoxyacetic Acid – Molecular Mechanisms. *Polish J. of Environ. Stud.* Vol. 15, No. 3 (2006), pp. 365-374, ISSN 1230-1485

Charles, J.M.; Bond, D.M., Jeffries, T.K., Yano, B.L., Stott, W.T., Johnson, K.A., Cunny, H.C., Wilson, R.D. & Bus, J.S. (1996a). Chronic dietary toxicity/oncogenicity studies on 2,4- dichlorophenoxyacetic acid in rodents. *Fundam. Appl. Toxicol.,* Vol. 33, No.2, (October 1996), pp. 166-172, ISSN 0272-0590

Charles, J.M.; Cunny, H.C., Wilson, R.D. & Bus, J.S. (1996b). Comparative subchronic studies on 2,4-dichlorophenoxyacetic acid, amine and ester in rats. *Fundam. Appl. Toxicol.,* Vol. 33, No.2, pp. 161-165, ISSN 0272-0590

Charles, J.M.; Cunny, H.C., Wilson, R.D., Ivett, J.L., Murli, H., Bus, J.S., & Gollapudi, B. (1999). In vivo micronucleus assays on 2,4-dichlorophenoxyacetic acid and its derivatives. *Mutat. Res.*, Vol. 444, No.1, (July 1999), pp. 227-234, ISSN 1383-5718

Chhabra, R. S.; Herbert, R. A., Roycroft, J. H., Chou, B., Miller, R. A. & Renne, R. A. (1998). Carcinogenesis Studies of Tetrahydrofuran Vapors in Rats and Mice. *Toxicological sciences*, Vol.41, pp. 183-188, ISSN 1096-6080

Cristaldi, M.; Ieradi, L.A., Mascanzoni, D. & Mattei, T. (1991). Environmental impact of the Chernobyl accident: mutagenesis in bank voles from Sweden. *Int. J. Radiat Biol.* Vol. 59, No.1, (January 1991), pp. 31–40, ISSN 0955-3002

CSGMT. (1992). Micronucleus test with mouse peripheral blood erythrocytes by acridine orange supra vital staining: The summary report of the 5th collaborative study by CSGMT/JEMS: MMS. The Collaborative Study Group for the Micronucleus Test. *Mutat Res*, Vol.278, No.2-3, (February-March 1992), pp. 83-98, ISSN 0027-5107

Cunningham, W.P. & Saigo, B.W. (1997). *Environmental science: A global concern*, p: 389, 4th ed. WMC Brown Publisher, ISBN 978-0697391520, New York.

Damek-Poprawa, M. & Sawicka-Kapusta, K. (2003). Damage to the liver, kidney, and testis with reference to burden of heavy metals in yellow-necked mice from areas around steelworks and zinc smelters in Poland. *Toxicology*, Vol.186, No.1-2, (April 2005), pp. 1-10, ISSN 0300-483X

de Souza Bueno, A.M.; de Bragança Pereira, C.A. & Rabello-Gay, M.N. (2000). Environmental Genotoxicity Evaluation Using Cytogenetic End Points in Wild Rodents. *Environ Health Perspect*, Vol.108, No.12, (December 2000), pp. 1165-1169, ISSN 0091-6765

Devi, K.D.; Banu, B.S., Grover, P. & Jamil, K. (2000). Genotoxic effect of lead nitrate on mice using SCGE (comet assay). *Toxicology*, Vol.145, No. 2-3, (April 2000), pp. 195–201, ISSN 0300-483X

Dhir, H.; Roy, A.K. & Sharma, A. (1993). Relative efficiency of Phyllanthus emblica fruit extract and ascorbic acid in modifying lead and aluminium-induced sister-chromatid exchanges in mouse bone marrow. *Environ Mol Mutagen*, Vol.21, No.3, (July 2006), pp. 229–236, ISSN 1098-2280

Ferreyra, H.; Romano, M. & Uhart, M. (2009). Recent and chronic exposure of wild ducks to lead in human-modified wetlands in Santa Fe Province, Argentina. *Journal of wildlife diseases*, Vol.45, No.3, (July 2009), pp. 823–827, ISSN 0090-3558

Gamer, A.O.; Jaeckh, R., Leibold, T., Kaufman, W., Gembardt, C., Bahnemann, R. & vonRavenzwaay B. (2002). Investigations on cell proliferation and enzyme induction in male rat kidney and female mouse liver caused by tetrahydrofuran. *Toxicological Sciences*, Vol.70, No.1, (November 2002), pp. 140-149, ISSN 1096-6080

Gandhi, R.; Wandji, S. & Snedeker, S. (2000). Critical evaluation of cancer risk from 2,4-D. *Rev. Environ. Contam. Toxicol.*, Vol.167, No.1, pp. 1-33, ISSN 0179-5953

Gerasimova, Ts. & Topashka-Ancheva, M. (2010). Experimental data for chromosome fragility in small mammal species (Rodentia, mammalia). *Comptes rendus de l'Acad_emie bulgare des Sciences*, Vol.63, No 2, (October 2009), pp. 277-284, ISSN 1310-1331

Gonzalez, M.; Soloneski, S., Reigosa, M.A. & Larramendy, M.L. (2005). Genotoxicity of the herbicide 2,4-dichlorophenoxyacetic and a commercial formulation, 2,4-dichlorophenoxyacetic acid dimethylamine salt. I. Evaluation of DNA damage and cytotoxic endpoints in Chinese hamster ovary (CHO) cells. *Toxicology in Vitro*, Vol.19, No.2, (March 2005), pp. 289-297, ISSN 0887-2333

Gosselin, R. E.; Hodge, H. C, Smith, R. P., & Gleason, M. N. (1976). *Clinical Toxicology of Commercial Products. Acute Poisoning*, 4th ed., ISBN 0683036319, Williams and Wilkins, Baltimore, MD.

Goyer, R.A. (1993). Lead toxicity: current concerns. *Environ. Health Perspect.*, Vol.100, (April 1993), pp. 177–187, ISSN 00916765

Gyrd-Hansen, N. & Dalgaard-Mikkelsen, S. (1974). The effect of phenoxyherbicides on the hatchability of eggs and the viability of chicks. *Acta Pharmacol. Toxicol.*, Vol.35, No.4, (October 1974), pp. 300-308, ISSN 0001-6683

Hagmar, L.; Stromberg, U., Bonassi, S., Hansteen, I.L., Knudsen, L.E., Lindholm, C. & Norppa, H. (2004). Impact of types of lymphocyte chromosomal aberrations on human cancer risk: results from Nordic and Italian cohorts. *Cancer Res.* Vol.64, No.6, (Mart 2004), pp. 2258-2263, ISSN 1538-7445

Hansen, W.H.; Quaife, M.L., Habermann, R.T. & Fitzhugh, O.G. (1971). Chronic toxicity of 2,4-dichlorophenoxyacetic acid in rats and dogs. *Toxicol. Appl. Pharmacol.*, Vol.20, No.1, (September 1994), pp. 122-129, ISSN 0041-008X

Hayes, H.M.; Tarone, R.E., Cantor, K.P., Jessen, C.R., McCurnin, D.M. & Richardson, R.C. (1991). Case-control study of canine malignant lymphoma: Positive association with dog owner's use of 2,4-dichlorophenoxyacetic acid herbicides. *J. Natl Cancer Inst.*, Vol. 83, No.17, (September 1991), pp. 1226-1231, ISSN 0027-8874

Heppner, C.W. & Schlatter, J.R. (2007). Food Additives & Contaminants: Part A: Chemistry, Analysis, Control, Exposure & Risk Assessment. Vol. 24, Issue S1, (September 2007), 114 – 121, ISSN 0265-203X.

Holland. N.T.; Duramad, P., Rothman, N., Figgs, L.W., Blair, A., Hubbard, A. & Smith, M.T. (2002). Micronucleus frequency and proliferation in human lymphocytes after exposure to herbicide 2,4-dichlorophenoxyacetic acid in vitro and in vivo. *Mutat Res.*, Vol.521, No.1-2, (August 2002), pp. 165-178, ISSN 1383-5718

IARC. (1987). *IARC Monographs on the Evaluation of Carcinogenic Risks to Humans, Supplement 6, Genetic and Related Effects: An Updating of Selected IARC Monographs from Volumes 1 to 42*, IARC Press, ISBN 92 832 1409 9, Lyon, pp. 351-354.

Ieradi, L.A.; Zima, J., Allegra, F., Kotlanova, E., Campanella, .L, Grossi, R. & Cristaldi, M. (2003). Evaluation of genotoxic damage in wild rodents from a polluted area in the Czech Republic. *Folia Zool.* Vol.52, No.1, (July 2002), pp. 57-66, ISSN 0139-7893

Jagetia, G.C. & Aruna, R. (1998). Effect of various concentrations of lead nitrate on the induction of micronuclei in mouse bone marrow. *Mutation Research*, Vol.415, No. 1-2, (July 1998), pp. 131–137, ISSN 1383-5718

Jena, G. & Bhunya, S. (1995). Use of chick, Gallus domesticus, as an in vivo model for the study of chromosome aberrations: A study with Mitomycin C and probable location of a 'hot spot'. *Mutation Research/ Environmental Mutagenesis and Related Subjects*, Vol.334, No.2, (April 1995), pp. 167–174, ISSN 1383-5718

Jin, Y.; Liao, Y., Lu, C., Li, G., Yu, F., Zhi, X., Xu, J., Liu, S., Liu, M. & Yang, J. (2006) Health effects of children aged 3–6 years induced by environmental lead exposure. *Ecotoxicol. Environ. Safety*, Vol. 63, No.2, (February 2006), pp. 313–317, ISSN 0147-6513

Karaivanova, M.; Koleva, M., Momekov, G., Kostadinov, I. & Delev, D. (2008). Toxic subsatances and intoxications, In: *Xenobiotics. Toxicity, preventive and therapeutic strategies.* Edited by Prof. Dr. M. Karaivanova, MD, First Edition, pp 311, Publ. by Softtreyd, ISBN 9789543340767, Sofia.

Katahira, T.; Teramoto, K. & Horiguchi, S. (1982). Experimental studies on the acute toxicity of tetrahyrofuran in animals. *Sangyo igaku Japanese journal of industrial health,* Vol. 24, No.4, (July 1982), 373-378, ISSN 0047-1879

Kipling, D.; Wilson, H.E., Mitchell, A.R., Teylor, B.A. & Cooke, H.J. (1994). Mouse centromeric mapping using oligonucleotide probe that detect variants of the minor satellite, *Chromosoma,* Vol.103, No.1, (March 1994), 46-55, ISSN 0009-5915

Kovalova, O. & Glazko, T. (2006). Radiation risk estimates in normal and emergency situations, In: *NATO security through science series – B: Physics and Biophysics,* Cigna, A. A.,Durante, M. (Eds.), pp. 95-100, Springer, ISBN 1-4020-4954-4

Lightfoot, T. & Yeager, J. (2008). Pet bird toxicity and related environmental concerns. The veterinary clinics of North America. *Exotic animal practice,* Vol. 11, No.2, (May 2008), pp. 229-259, ISSN 1094-9194

Ma, W.C. (1996). Lead in mammals. In: *Environmental Contaminants in Wildlife: Interpreting Tissue Concentrations,* W. N. Beyer, G. H. Heinz and A. W. Redmon-Norwood (Eds.), (pp. 281-296), SETAC Special Publication Series. Lewis Publishers, Boca Raton, ISBN 978-1566700719, Florida.

Marques, C.C.; Nunes, A.C., Pinheiro, T., Lopes, P.A., Santos, M.C., Viegas-Crespo, A.M., Ramalhinho, M.G. & Mathias, M.L. (2006) An assessment of time-dependent effects of lead exposure in Algerian mice (*Mus spretus*) using different methodological approaches. *Biol. Trace Elem. Res.,* Vol.109, No.1, (January 2009), pp. 75-90, ISSN 0163-4984

Mateuca, R.; Lombaert, N., Aka, P.V., Decordier, I. & Kirsch-Volders, M. (2006). Chromosomal changes: induction, detection methods and applicability in human monitoring. *Biochimie,* Vol.88, No.11, (November 2006), pp. 1515-1531, ISSN 0300-9084

Matthey, R. (1936). La formule chromosomiale et les heterochromosomes chez les Apodemus europeens, *Z. Zellforsch. Mirkosk. Anat.,* vol. 25, pp. 501–519.

Metcheva, R.; S. Teodorova & Topashka – Ancheva, M. (2003). A comparative analysis of the heavy metal loading of small mammals in different regions of Bulgaria I: monitoring points and bioaccumulation features. *Ecotoxicological research and enviromental safety,* Vol.54, No.2, (February 2003), pp. 176-187, ISSN 0147-6513

Metcheva, R.; Teodorova. S. & Topashka-Ancheva, M. (2001). A comparative analysis of the heavy metals and toxic elements loading indicated by small mammals in different Bulgarian regions. *Acta Zool Bulg.,* J.P. Carbonnel et J.N. Stamenov (Eds.), Vol.53, No.1, pp. 61-80, Sofia: Inst. for Nuclear Research and Nuclear Energy, ISSN 0324-0770, Sofia

Metcheva, R.; Topashka-Ancheva, M., Beltcheva, M., Artinian, A. & Nikolova, E. (1996). Population and biological characteristics of different monitor species small mammals from the region of Beli Iskar artificial dam in National park Rila. In: *Observatoire de Montagne de Moussala OM2,* Vol. 4, pp. 168 -176, ISBN 954-90025-4-3

Milton, A.; Cooke, J.A. & Johnson, M.S. (2003). Accumulation of lead, zinc and cadmium in a wild population of *Clethrionomys glareolus* from an abandoned lead mine. *Arch. Environ. Contam. Toxicol.* Vol.44, No.3, (April 2003), pp. 405-411, ISSN 0090-4341

Mitsainas, G.P.; Tryfonopoulos, G.A., Thanou, E.G. Bisa, R., Fraguedakis-Tsolis, S.E. & Chondropoulos, Basilios, P. (2009). New data on the distribution of *Mus spicilegus* Petenyi, 1882 (Rodentia, Muridae) and adistinct mtDNA lineage in the southern Balkans. *Mamm. biol.*, Vol. 74, No.5, (September 2009), pp. 351–360, ISSN 1616-5047

Mohammed-Brahim, B.; Buchet, J.P. & Lauwerys, R. (1985). Erythrocyte pyrimidine 5′-nucleotidase activity in workers exposed to lead, mercury or cadmium. *Int Arch Occup Environ Health, Vol.* 55, No. 3, pp. 247–252, ISSN 0340-0131

Natarajan, A.T. (1993). Mechanisms for induction of mutations and chromosome alterations. *Environmental Health Perspectives Supplements*, Vol.101, (Suppl.3), (October 1993), pp. 225-229, ISSN 0091-6765

Nayak, B.N.; Ray, M., Persaud, T.V.N. & Nigli, M. (1989). Relationship of embryotoxicity to genotoxicity of lead nitrate in mice. *Exp. Pathol.*, Vo.36, No.2, pp. 65-73, ISSN 0232-1513

NRDC (Earth's Best Defence). (2008). Natural resources defense council's petition to revoke all tolerances and cancel all registrations for the pesticide 2,4 D. (November 2008), pp. 1-14.

NTP. (1998). *Toxicology and carcinogenesis studies of tetrahydrofuran (CAS No. 109-99-9) in F344/N rats and B6C3F1 mice.* Public Health Service, U.S. Department of Health and Human Services; NTP TR- 475.

O'Brien, D.J.; Kaneene, J.B. & Poppenga, R,H. (1993). The use of mammals as sentinelsfor human exposure to toxic contaminants in the environment. *EnvironHealth Perspect.*, Vol.99, (March 1993), pp. 351-368, ISSN 0091-6765

Patil, A.J.; Bhagwat, V.R., Patil, J.A., Dongre, N.N., Ambekar, J.G. & Das, K.K. (2006) Biochemical aspects of lead exposure in silver jewelry workers in western Maharashtra (India). *J. Basic. Clin. Physiol. Pharmacol.*, Vol.17, No.4, pp. 213–129, ISSN 2191-0286

Pfeiffer, P.; Goedecke, W. & Obe, G. (2000). Mechanisms of DNA double-strand repair and their potential to induce chromosomal aberrations. *Mutagenesis*, Vol.15, No. 4, pp. 289-302, ISSN 0267-8357

Preston, R.J.; Dean, B., Galloway, S., Holden, H., McFee, A.F., Sheldy, M. (1987). Mammalian in vivo cytogenetic assay analysis of chromosome aberrations in bone marrow cells. *Mutation Research/Genetic Toxicology*, Vol.189, pp. 157–165, ISSN 1383-5718

Reynolds, P.M.; Reif, J.S., Ramsdell, H.S. & Tessari J.D. (1994). Canine exposure to herbicide-treated lawns and urinary excretion of 2,4-dichlorophenoxyacetic acid. *Cancer Epidemiology, Biomarkers & Prevention*, Vol.3, No.3, (April-May 1994), pp. 233-237, ISSN 1055-996

Rosso, S.B; Garcia, G.B., Madariaga, M.J., Evangelista de Duffard, A.M., & Duffard, R.O. (2000). 2,4-Dichlorophenoxyacetic acid in developing rats alters behaviour, myelination and regions brain gangliosides pattern. *Neurotoxicol.* Vol.21, No.1-2, (February-April 2000), pp. 155-164, ISSN 0161-813X

Roy, N.K. & Rossman, T.G. (1992). Mutagenesis and comutagenesis by lead compounds. *Mutation Res.*, Vol.298, No.2, (December 1992), pp. 97-103, ISSN 1383-5718

Sánchez-Chardi; A., Peñarroja-Matutano, C., Oliveira Ribeiro, C.A. & Nadal, J. (2007). Bioaccumulation of metals and effects of a landfill in small mammals. Part II. The wood mouse, *Apodemus sylvaticus. Chemosphere*, Vol.70, No.1, (November 2007), pp. 101-109, ISSN 0045-6535

Shaik, A.P.; Sankar, S.; Ready, S.C.; Das, P.G.; Jamil, K. (2006). Lead-induced genotoxicity in lymphocytes from peripheral blood samples of humans: in vitro studies. *Drug and Chemical Toxicology,*Vol. 29, *No.*1, (February 2006), pp. 111-124, ISSN 0148-0545

Sharma, R.K.; Jacobson-Kram, D., Lemmon, M., Bakke, J., Galperin, I. & Blazak, W.F. (1985). Sister chromatid exchange and cell replication kinetics in fetal and maternal cells after treatment with chemical teratogens. *Mutat Res.*, Vol.158, No.3, pp. 217–231, ISSN 1383-5718

Shore, R.F. & Douben, P.E.T. (1994). The ecotoxicological significance of cadmium intake and residues in terrestrial small mammals. *Ecotoxicol Environ Saf* 1994; Vol.29, No.1, (October 1994), pp. 101–112, ISSN 0147-6513

Shore, R.F. & Rattner, B.A. (March 2001).*Ecotoxicology of wild mammals* (1st edition), John Wiley & Sons, ISBN 978-0-471-97429-1, London

Sierra Club of Canada. (2005). Overview of the toxic effects of 2,4-D. Prepared by: 412-1 Nicholas St. Ottawa, ON.

Sorsa, M., Wilbourn, J. & Vainio, H. (1992). Human cytogenetic damage as a predictor of cancer risk, In: *Mechanisms of Carcinogenesis in Risk Identification,* Vainio H., Magee P.H., McGregor D.B., McMichael A.J. (Eds.) pp. 543-554, IARC Scientific Publication no. 116 (WHO), ISBN 978-9283221166, Lyons and International Agency for Research on Cancer, New York

Sorsa, M.; Ojajärvi, A. & Salomaa, S. (1990). Cytogenetic surveillance of workers exposed to genotoxic chemicals: Preliminary experiences from a prospective cancer study in a cytogenetic cohort. Teratog Carcinog Mutagen., Vol.10, No.3, pp. 215-221, ISSN 0270-3211

Testa, A.; Ranaldi, R., Carpineto, L., Pacchierotti, F., Tirindelli, D., Fabiani, L., Giuliani. A.R., Urso, M., Rossini, A., Materazzo, F., Petyx, M. & Leoni, V. (2002). Cytogenetic biomonitoring of workers from laboratories of clinical analyses occupationally exposed to chemicals *Mutation Research*, Vol.520, No.1-2, (September 2002), pp. 73–82, ISSN 1383-5718

Tomasz, M.; Lipman, R., Chowdary, D., Pawlak, J., Verdine, G.L. & Nakanishi, K. (1987). Isolation and structure of a covalent cross-link adduct between mitomycin C and DNA. *Science*, Vol.235, No.4793, (March 1987), pp. 1204-1208, ISSN 0036-8075

Topashka-Ancheva; M., Metcheva, R. & S. Teodorova. (2003). A comperative analyses of the heavy metals loading of small mammals in different Bulgarian Regions. II. Chromosomal aberrations and blood pathology. *Ecotoxicology and Environmental Safety*, Vol 54, No.2, (February 2003), pp. 188 – 193, ISSN 0147-6513

Topashka-Ancheva, M. & Metcheva, R. (1999). Bioaccumulation of heavy metals and chromosome aberrations in small mammals from industrially polluted region in Bulgaria. *Contr. zoogeogr Ecol Eastern Mediterr. Region*, Vol.1, (Suppl.), pp. 69-74.

Topashka-Ancheva, M. & Teodorova, S.E. (2010). Toxic effects of lead and cadmium as industrial pollutants on the chromosome structure in model mammalian species (Chapter 7). In: *Impact, Monitoring and Management of Environmental Pollution*. El Nemr A. (Ed.), pp. 133-155, Nova Science Publishers Inc. ISBN 978-1-60876-487-7, New York

Turkula, T.E., & Jalal, S.M. (1985). Increased rates of sister chromatid exchanges induced by the herbicide 2,4-D. *J. Hered.*, Vol. 76, No.3, (Maj-June 1985) pp. 213-214, ISSN 0022-1503

Valverde, M.; Fortoul, T.I., Diaz-Barriga, F., Mejia, J. & del Castillo, E.R. (2002). Genotoxicity induced in CD-1 mice by inhaled lead: differential organ response. *Mutagenesis,* Vol.17, No.1, (January 2002), pp. 55-61, ISSN 0267-8357

Vanio, H. & Sorsa, M. (1991). Role of Cytogenetic Surveillance to Assess Exposure to Carcinogens, In: *Methods for Assessing Exposure of Human and Non-Human Biota.* R.G. Tardiff and B. Goldstein (Eds) SCOPE 1991, pp. 309-322, Published by John Wiley & Sons LId, ISBN 0 471 92954 9, New York

Veličković, M. (2004). Chromosomal aberrancy and the level of fluctuating asymmetry in black-striped mouse (*Apodemus agrarius*): effects of disturbed environment. *Hereditas,* Vol.140, No.2, (April 2004), pp. 112–122, ISSN 0018-0661

Venkov, P.; M. Topashka-Ancheva, M. Georgieva, V. Alexieva and E. Karanov. (2000). Genotoxic effect of substituted phenoxyacetic acids. *Archives of Toxicology,* Vol. 74, N 9, (November 2000), pp. 560-566, ISSN 0340-5761

Water Hyacinth Control Program. (September 2009). Hazards and Hazardous Materials Impacts Assessment, In: *Programmatic Environmental Impact Report,* Sacramento, California Department of Boating and Waterways R-17, Vol.1, Chapters 1 to 7, pp. 1- 304.

Zima J.& Král, B. (1984). Karyotypes of European mammals II. *Acta Sc. Nat. Brno,* Vol.18, No.8, pp. 1–62, ISSN 0032-8758

Zima, J. (1985). Chromosome aberrations in populations of the common vole (*Microtus arvalis*) from certain regions in Czechoslovakia. *Ekologia CSFR,* Vol.4, No.3, pp. 241-249, ISSN 0862-9129

Zima, J. (2004). Karyotype variation in mammals of the Balkan Peninsula. In: *Balkan Biodiversity: Pattern and process in the European hotspot,* Griffiths H.I., Krystufek B. & Reed K.M. (eds), pp. 109-133, Springer-Verlag, ISBN 9781402028533, New York

Permissions

The contributors of this book come from diverse backgrounds, making this book a truly international effort. This book will bring forth new frontiers with its revolutionizing research information and detailed analysis of the nascent developments around the world.

We would like to thank Dr. Ghousia Begum, for lending his expertise to make the book truly unique. He has played a crucial role in the development of this book. Without his invaluable contribution this book wouldn't have been possible. He has made vital efforts to compile up to date information on the varied aspects of this subject to make this book a valuable addition to the collection of many professionals and students.

This book was conceptualized with the vision of imparting up-to-date information and advanced data in this field. To ensure the same, a matchless editorial board was set up. Every individual on the board went through rigorous rounds of assessment to prove their worth. After which they invested a large part of their time researching and compiling the most relevant data for our readers. Conferences and sessions were held from time to time between the editorial board and the contributing authors to present the data in the most comprehensible form. The editorial team has worked tirelessly to provide valuable and valid information to help people across the globe.

Every chapter published in this book has been scrutinized by our experts. Their significance has been extensively debated. The topics covered herein carry significant findings which will fuel the growth of the discipline. They may even be implemented as practical applications or may be referred to as a beginning point for another development. Chapters in this book were first published by InTech; hereby published with permission under the Creative Commons Attribution License or equivalent.

The editorial board has been involved in producing this book since its inception. They have spent rigorous hours researching and exploring the diverse topics which have resulted in the successful publishing of this book. They have passed on their knowledge of decades through this book. To expedite this challenging task, the publisher supported the team at every step. A small team of assistant editors was also appointed to further simplify the editing procedure and attain best results for the readers.

Our editorial team has been hand-picked from every corner of the world. Their multi-ethnicity adds dynamic inputs to the discussions which result in innovative outcomes. These outcomes are then further discussed with the researchers and contributors who give their valuable feedback and opinion regarding the same. The feedback is then collaborated with the researches and they are edited in a comprehensive manner to aid the understanding of the subject.

Apart from the editorial board, the designing team has also invested a significant amount of their time in understanding the subject and creating the most relevant covers. They scrutinized every image to scout for the most suitable representation of the subject and create an appropriate cover for the book.

The publishing team has been involved in this book since its early stages. They were actively engaged in every process, be it collecting the data, connecting with the contributors or procuring relevant information. The team has been an ardent support to the editorial, designing and production team. Their endless efforts to recruit the best for this project, has resulted in the accomplishment of this book. They are a veteran in the field of academics and their pool of knowledge is as vast as their experience in printing. Their expertise and guidance has proved useful at every step. Their uncompromising quality standards have made this book an exceptional effort. Their encouragement from time to time has been an inspiration for everyone.

The publisher and the editorial board hope that this book will prove to be a valuable piece of knowledge for researchers, students, practitioners and scholars across the globe.

List of Contributors

Elke Jurandy Bran Nogueira Cardoso and Paulo Roger Lopes Alves
Universidade de São Paulo - Escola Superior de Agriculura "Luiz de Queiroz", Brazil

Sabria Barka
Research Unit of Marine and Environmental Toxicology, UR 09-03, University of Sfax, Institut Supérieur de Biotechnologie de Monastir, Tunisia

Sara Pires, João Lopes, Inês Nunes and Elvira Gaspar
CQFB-REQUIMTE/Departamento de Química/Faculdade de Ciências e Tecnologia/ Universidade Nova de Lisboa, Portugal

Pane Luigi, Agrone Chiara, Giacco Elisabetta, Somà Alessandra and Mariottini Gian Luigi
DIP.TE.RIS, University of Genova, Genova, Italy

Petr Dvorak and Jiri Vitek
University of Veterinary and Pharmaceutical Sciences, Czech Republic

Katarina Benova
University of Veterinary Medicine and Pharmacy, Slovak Republic

Sumer Aras, Semra Soydam Aydin, Didem Aksoy Körpe and Çiğdem Dönmez
Ankara University, Turkey

Margarita Topashka-Ancheva and Tsvetelina Gerasimova
Institute of Biodiversity and Ecosystem Research, Bulgarian Academy of Sciences, Sofia, Bulgaria

Printed in the USA
CPSIA information can be obtained
at www.ICGtesting.com
JSHW011334221024
72173JS00003B/156